Obstetric and Gynecologic Hospitalists and Laborists

Editors

AMY VANBLARICOM
BRIGID MCCUE

OBSTETRICS AND GYNECOLOGY CLINICS OF NORTH AMERICA

www.obgyn.theclinics.com

Consulting Editor
WILLIAM F. RAYBURN

September 2024 • Volume 51 • Number 3

ELSEVIER

1600 John F. Kennedy Boulevard • Suite 1800 • Philadelphia, Pennsylvania, 19103-2899

http://www.theclinics.com

OBSTETRICS AND GYNECOLOGY CLINICS OF NORTH AMERICA Volume 51 Number 3
September 2024 ISSN 0889-8545, ISBN-13: 978-0-443-24642-5

Editor: Kerry Holland
Developmental Editor: Saswoti Nath

Obstetrics and Gynecology Clinics (ISSN 0889-8545) is published quarterly by Elsevier Inc., 360 Park Avenue South, New York, NY 10010-1710. Months of issue are March, June, September, and December. Periodicals postage paid at New York, NY, and additional mailing offices. Subscription price per year is $355.00 (US individuals), $100.00 (US students), $428.00 (Canadian individuals), $100.00 (Canadian students), $497.00 (international individuals), $956.00 (international institutions), and $225.00 (international students). For institutional access pricing please contact Customer Service via the contact information below. To receive student/resident rate, orders must be accompanied by name of affiliated institution, date of term, and the signature of program/residency coordinator on institution letterhead. Orders will be billed at individual rate until proof of status is received. Foreign air speed delivery is included in all *Clinics* subscription prices. All prices are subject to change without notice. Orders, claims, and journal inquiries: Please visit our Support Hub page https://service.elsevier.com for assistance.

Reprints. For copies of 100 or more of articles in this publication, please contact the Commercial Reprints Department, Elsevier Inc., 360 Park Avenue South, New York, New York 10010-1710. Tel.: 212-633-3874; Fax: 212-633-3820; E-mail: reprints@elsevier.com.

Obstetrics and Gynecology Clinics of North America is also published in Spanish by McGraw-Hill Interamericana Editores S.A., P.O. Box 5-237, 06500, Mexico; in Portuguese by Reichmann and Affonso Editores, Rio de Janeiro, Brazil; and in Greek by Paschalidis Medical Publications, Athens, Greece.

Obstetrics and Gynecology Clinics of North America is covered in MEDLINE/PubMed (Index Medicus), Excerpta Medica, Current Concepts/Clinical Medicine, Science Citation Index, BIOSIS, CINAHL, and ISI/BIOMED.

Contributors

CONSULTING EDITOR

WILLIAM F. RAYBURN, MD, MBA
Affiliate Professor, Department of Obstetrics and Gynecology and College of Graduate Studies, Medical University of South Carolina, Charleston, South Carolina; Emeritus Distinguished Professor, Department of Obstetrics and Gynecology, University of New Mexico School of Medicine, Albuquerque, New Mexico

EDITORS

AMY VANBLARICOM, MD
Chief Clinical Officer, Obstetrics and Gynecology, OB Hospitalist Group, Seattle, Washington; Chief Clinical Officer, OB Hospitalist Group, Greenville, South Carolina

BRIGID McCUE, MD, PhD, FACOG
Director OB/GYN Hospitalist Fellowship, OB/GYN Hospitalist, Assistant Professor, Department of Obstetrics and Gynecology, South Shore University Hospital, Zucker School of Medicine at Hofstra/Northwell, Bay Shore, New York

AUTHORS

MEGAN R. ANSBRO, MD, PhD
Cleveland Clinic Foundation, Obstetric and Gynecologic Institute, Cleveland, Ohio

SARAH L. BRADLEY, MD
UW Health Northern Illinois, Rockford, Illinois

JOSHUA S. BRUNTON, DO
Department of Obstetrics and Gynecology, Mayo Clinic, Rochester, Minnesota

JENNIFER R. BUTLER, MD
Clinical Professor of Medicine, University of California Irvine, Orange, California

SARA CARRANCO, MD
Department of Obstetrics and Gynecology, Baylor College of Medicine, Houston, Texas

SARAH N. CROSS, MD
Associate Professor, Division of Maternal Fetal Medicine, Department of Obstetrics, Gynecology and Reproductive Sciences, Yale School of Medicine, New Haven, Connecticut

EESHA DAVE, MD
Instructor, Division of Maternal Fetal Medicine, Department of Obstetrics, Gynecology and Reproductive Sciences, Yale School of Medicine, New Haven, Connecticut

JULIANNE DEMARTINO, MD, FACOG
OB/GYN Hospitalist, OB Hospitalist Education Director, Obstetric Simulation Director, University Hospitals Cleveland, Case Western Reserve University

JENNIFER L. EATON, DO
Assistant Professor of Reproductive Biology, Cleveland Clinic Lerner College of Medicine, Case Western Reserve University, Cleveland Clinic, Obstetrics and Gynecology Institute, Cleveland, Ohio

VICTORIA N. FERRENTINO, Esq
Ferrentino + Brotz, Tampa, Florida

JOY FEST, MD
Department of Obstetrics and Gynecology, South Shore University Hospital, Zucker School of Medicine at Hofstra/Northwell, Bay Shore, New York

ALYSSA K. GONZALEZ, MD
Resident Physician, University of California Irvine, Orange, California

ANTHONY GRANDELIS, MD
Director of OB/GYN Medical Education, Department of Obstetrics and Gynecology, Columbia University, New York, New York

SHEILA HILL, MD
Director, Division of Hospitalist Medicine, Assistant Professor, Department of Obstetrics & Gynecology, Baylor College of Medicine, Texas Children's Pavilion for Women, Houston, Texas

MONIQUE YODER KATSUKI, MD, MPH, FACOG
OB/GYN Hospitalist, Cleveland Clinic Foundation, Obstetric and Gynecologic Institute; Assistant Professor, OB/GYN and Reproductive Biology, Cleveland Clinic Lerner College of Medicine, Case Western Reserve University, Cleveland, Ohio

KATHERINE S. KOHARI, MD
Associate Director, Fetal Care Center, Medical Director, Outpatient Services, Division of Maternal Fetal Medicine, Assistant Professor, Department of Obstetrics, Gynecology and Reproductive Sciences, Yale School of Medicine, New Haven, Connecticut

ANDREA LUGOMORALES, MD
Department of Obstetrics and Gynecology, Baylor College of Medicine, Houston, Texas

BRIGID McCUE, MD, PhD, FACOG
Director OB/GYN Hospitalist Fellowship, OB/GYN Hospitalist, Assistant Professor, Department of Obstetrics and Gynecology, South Shore University Hospital, Zucker School of Medicine at
Hofstra/Northwell, Bay Shore, New York

LISBETH M. McKINNON, MD, FACOG
Director of OB/GYN Hospitalists, Overlake Medical Center, Bellevue, Washington; Market Medical Director, OB-Hospitalist Group, Greenville, South Carolina

KIM M. PUTERBAUGH, MD
SSM Health, Saint Anthony Hospital, Oklahoma City, Oklahoma

WILLIAM F. RAYBURN, MD, MBA
Affiliate Professor, Department of Obstetrics and Gynecology and College of Graduate Studies, Medical University of South Carolina, Charleston, South Carolina; Emeritus Distinguished Professor, Department of Obstetrics and Gynecology, University of New Mexico School of Medicine, Albuquerque, New Mexico

EILEEN M. REARDON, MD, FACOG
OB/GYN Hospitalist, Intermountain Health, Peaks Region, Denver, Colorado

VICKI R. REED, MD
Clinical Assistant Professor of Reproductive Biology, Cleveland Clinic Lerner College of Medicine, Case Western Reserve University, Cleveland Clinic, Obstetrics and Gynecology Institute, Cleveland, Ohio

MARK N. SIMON, MD, MMM
Chief Medical Officer, OB Hospitalist Group, Greenville, South Carolina

VASILIKI TATSIS, MD, MS, MBA
Professor, Division Chief - OB/GYN Hospital Medicine, Fellowship Director - OB/GYN Hospital Medicine Department of Obstetrics, Gynecology, and Reproductive Sciences, University of California, San Francisco, San Francisco, California

VANESSA E. TORBENSON, MD
Department of Obstetrics and Gynecology, Mayo Clinic, Rochester, Minnesota

AMY VANBLARICOM, MD
Chief Clinical Officer, Obstetrics and Gynecology, OB Hospitalist Group, Seattle, Washington; Chief Clinical Officer, OB Hospitalist Group, Greenville, South Carolina

LARRY VELTMAN, MD, FACOG, CPHRM, DFASHRM
Portland, Oregon

WILLIAM F. RAYBURN, MD, MBA

Associate Professor, Department of Obstetrics and Gynecology and College of Graduate Studies, Medical University of South Carolina, Charleston, South Carolina; Emeritus Distinguished Professor, Department of Obstetrics and Gynecology, University of New Mexico School of Medicine, Albuquerque, New Mexico

EILEEN M. REARDON, MD, FACOG

OB/GYN Hospitalist, Intermountain Health, Peaks Region, Denver, Colorado

VICKI R. REED, MD

Clinical Assistant Professor of Reproductive Biology, Cleveland Clinic Lerner College of Medicine, Case Western Reserve University, Cleveland Clinic, Cleveland; and OB/Gynecology Institute, Cleveland, Ohio

MARK N. SIMON, MD, MMM

Chief Medical Officer, OB Hospitalist Group, Greenville, South Carolina

VASILIKI TATSIS, MD, MS, MBA

Professor, Division Chief - OB GYN Hospitalist Medicine, Fellowship Director - OB/GYN Hospitalist Medicine, Department of Obstetrics, Gynecology and Reproductive Sciences, University of California, San Francisco, San Francisco, California

VANESSA E. TORBENSON, MD

Department of Obstetrics and Gynecology, Mayo Clinic, Rochester, Minnesota

AMY VANBLARICOM, MD

Chief Clinical Officer, Obstetrics and Gynecology, OB Hospitalist Group, Seattle, Washington; Chief Clinical Officer, OB Hospitalist Group, Greenville, South Carolina

LARRY VEITMAN, MD, FACOG, CPHRM, DFASHRM

Portland, Oregon

Contents

> As the field of obstetrics and gynecology (Ob/Gyn) evolves, the role of the Ob/Gyn hospitalists has become increasingly integrated into the framework of the specialty. Ob/Gyn hospitalists take on essential responsibilities as competent clinicians in emergent situations and as hospital leaders: maintaining standard of care, collaborating with community practitioners and care teams, promoting diversity, equity, and inclusion practices, and contributing to educational initiatives. The impact of the Ob/Gyn hospitalists is positive for patients, fellow clinicians, and institutions. As the field continues to change and the Ob/Gyn hospitalist develops as an established subspecialty, further research evaluating its role remains essential.

> Maternal mortality in the United States has risen steadily over the past 20 years. Several interventions including maternal mortality committees and safety bundles have been introduced to decrease the trend. Severe maternal morbidity is a more frequent occurrence related to maternal mortality and can be used to track interventions. Within safety bundles, the presence of well-trained on-site staff such as obstetrics and gynecology (OB/GYN) hospitalists is key to correct implementation. In this article, the authors review the role of OB/GYN hospitalists in specific diagnoses and the evidence present to date on OB/GYN hospitalists' role in decreasing severe maternal morbidity.

> Obstetrics and gynecologic hospitalists play a pivotal role in the evolution of perinatal care. Hospitalists improve patient safety by providing on-site, reliable, high-quality care. Hospitalists help to reduce the rates of unnecessary cesarean deliveries and increase the rates of vaginal deliveries.

The concept of a 24/7 in-house obstetrician, serving as an obstetrics and gynecology (Ob/Gyn) hospitalist, provides a safety-net for obstetric and gynecologic events that may need immediate intervention for a successful outcome. The addition of an Ob/Gyn hospitalist role in the perinatal department mitigates loss prevention, a key precept of risk management. Inherent in the role of the Ob/Gyn hospitalist are the important patient safety and risk management principles of layers of back-up, enhanced teamwork and communications, and immediate availability.

Creating and managing a successful obstetric and gynecologic (OB hospitalist) program requires careful attention to multiple aspects of the program. Appropriate policies and procedures need to be created. The clinical team needs to be selected and trained. Measurement of clinical and operational activity needs to be implemented and transparently shared with the team and the hospital partner. This all should be done with the hospital's goals for the program in mind and recognizing the type of clinical care that the hospital provides for obstetric patients in its community.

An obstetric emergency department (OBED) allows for timely, standardized and quality care by a clinician for pregnant patients presenting unscheduled to a hospital. Understanding the differences between a traditional labor and delivery triage model and an OBED are important in developing a successful, safe, and quality obstetric program that meets the needs of the community with appropriate resource allocation. The benefits in an OBED of every patient seen in a timely fashion by a clinician, and ultimately the impact on outcomes are noteworthy and should be considered when developing a labor and delivery unit.

Due to improved outcomes in clinical care, patient safety, and education, demand for OBGYN hospitalists is increasing. As a result, an OBGYN hospitalist fellowship was developed to train future leaders in OBGYN hospital medicine. This article is a discussion regarding the landscape of OBGYN hospitalist fellowships across the country. Utilizing information from program-specific Web sites, as well as discussions with past and present fellowship directors, this article summarizes key differences and similarities across programs, as well as reviews important considerations for those hoping to start a fellowship at their own institution.

care, teaching, research, and inpatient leadership. Primarily, they manage obstetric and gynecologic patients in the hospital, handling emergencies and providing urgent care. Hospitalists oversee the entire continuum of patient care, from the emergency department to post-acute follow-up. This model emphasizes the traditional academic attending physician's role, particularly that of the gynecologic hospitalist, who excels in acute inpatient obstetric and gynecologic medicine, advancing skills in urgent care and medical education, and ensuring quality and safety metrics.

Periviability for the Ob-Gyn Hospitalist   567

Eesha Dave, Katherine S. Kohari, and Sarah N. Cross

Periviable birth refers to births occurring between 20 0/7 and 25 6/7 weeks gestational age. Management of pregnant people and neonates during this fragile time depends on the clinical status, as well as the patient's wishes. Providers should be prepared to counsel patients at the cusp of viability, being mindful of the uncertainty of outcomes for these neonates. While it is important to incorporate the data on projected morbidity and mortality into one's counseling, shared-decision making is most essential to caring for these patients and optimizing outcomes for all.

OBSTETRICS AND GYNECOLOGY CLINICS

THE CLINICS ARE AVAILABLE ONLINE!
Access your subscription at:
www.theclinics.com

FORTHCOMING ISSUES

December 2024
Addressing Mental Health in Obstetrics and Gynecology
Iffath Abbasi Hoskins and Olumhense Mahdokht, Editors

March 2025
Pediatric and Adolescent Gynecology
Marc R. Laufer, Editor

June 2025
Updates in Family Planning
Rachel Flink-Bochacki and Lauren Thaxton, Editors

RECENT ISSUES

June 2024
Sexual Medicine for Obstetrician-Gynecologists
Monica M. Christmas and Andrew Robert Fisher, Editors

March 2024
Diversity, Equity, and Inclusion in Obstetrics and Gynecology
Versha Pleasant, Editor

December 2023
Reproductive Endocrinology and Infertility
Amanda J. Adeleye and Albaran Muasa Zamah, Editors

Foreword

The Obstetric and Gynecologic Hospitalist: An Established Practice Model Rather than a Concept

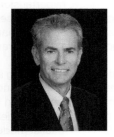

William F. Rayburn, MD, MBA
Consulting Editor

This quarter's issue of the *Obstetrics and Gynecology Clinics of North America* pertains to The Ob/Gyn Hospitalist. An obstetric and gynecologic (OB/GYN) hospitalist refers to an OB/GYN who has minimal outpatient and elective surgical responsibilities, and whose primary role is to care for hospitalized obstetric patients and to help manage obstetric emergencies that occur in the hospital. The Society for Maternal-Fetal Medicine and Society of OB/GYN Hospitalists have endorsed and reaffirmed the American College of Obstetricians and Gynecologists' Committee Opinions on Patient Safety and Quality Improvement and Obstetric Practices on The Obstetric and Gynecologic Hospitalist.

Our original issue about The OB/GYN Hospitalist was in 2015. Continued advancement led me to approach Dr Amy VanBlaricom and Dr Brigid McCue to prepare an update that is applicable to rural hospitals and urban tertiary care centers. The editors' positive response was tempered by the understanding to prepare an issue that best suited the readership. Their effort in completing this task led to a valuable contribution to our limited literature on the subject. The 31 expert authors prepared 13 articles that focused on a variety of subjects: severe maternal morbidity and mortality, safety and quality metrics, risk management, triage versus emergency department utilization, health care inequities, fellowship training, education, drills and simulations, crisis management, preterm labor and delivery, and gynecologic hospital needs.

In reviewing each article and references, I was impressed at how far the field has developed in the past decade. More has been undertaken to improve patient safety and professional satisfaction. Hospitals and OB/GYN hospitalist staffing companies

Obstet Gynecol Clin N Am 51 (2024) xiii–xv
https://doi.org/10.1016/j.ogc.2024.06.003
0889-8545/24/© 2024 Published by Elsevier Inc.

obgyn.theclinics.com

require participating physicians to achieve and maintain expertise in the many topics addressed in this issue. Hospitalists help manage the continuum of patient care, often from being seen in the triage area, monitoring them in hospital, and organizing post-acute care. Communication is more effective in many ways: patient handoffs, updates on progress, protocol development, and follow-up instructions with patients, nurses, and other health care providers.

Benefits with the OB/GYN hospitalist model would be in reducing certain undesired events (eg, high cesarean delivery rates, venous thromboembolism, inductions before 39 weeks), provider sleep deprivation or fatigue, and less standardized care. A hospitalist program may afford more autonomy for office-based physicians through coverage of their laboring patients, attending to rapidly delivering patients or urgencies (eg, worrisome fetal heart rate tracings, obstetric hemorrhage, hypertension), or when they are either in the middle of busy office hours or operative cases. Hospitalists in many practice models benefit from predictable schedules, fewer unanticipated clinical responsibilities, competitive compensation and benefits, and guaranteed time off.

Certain challenges mentioned in this issue deserve our attention when employing an OB/GYN hospitalist model. Hospitalists may have difficulty in maintaining competency in major gynecologic surgeries, and office-based OB/GYNs may be more limited in demonstrating continued competency in certain aspects of obstetric care. Patient satisfaction is likely either unaffected or improved with the OB/GYN hospitalist model, but additional research is needed. In collaboration with the hospital, a hospitalist needs to understand operating costs, attempt to affirm a manageable volume, and maintain their qualifications. Standardized protocols and clear communication channels must be periodically assessed and agreed upon by a multidisciplinary team.

Of particular interest to me is the training of OB/GYN hospitalists, since more are recent residency graduates who must be sufficiently trained. Hospitalists often supervise and teach students and residents, provide consultative and surgical support to certified nurse midwives and family physicians, and manage unassigned patients. More is known about candidates for positions as OB/GYN hospitalists because of refinements in documented training and experience appropriate for the management of the acute and potentially emergent clinical circumstances that may be encountered. There is a growing number of fellowship programs available for those seeking additional training in risk management, more effective teaching, and business development. Despite this, there is no subspecialty certification recognized at this time by the Accreditation Council on Graduate Medical Education or the American Board of Obstetrics and Gynecology...perhaps there may eventually be a "focused practice designation."

Progress in the OB/GYN hospitalist model continues to show not only promise but also stability with the potential to achieve benefits for obstetric patients, OB/GYN providers, and hospitals. I appreciate the efforts by Dr VanBlaricom, Dr McCue, and the many authors in sharing their experience relevant to inpatient practice settings. Topics addressed in this issue incorporate priorities that encompass essential core metrics for more optimal women's inpatient health care. Moving forward, more studies are needed to demonstrate the effect of care provided by OB/GYN hospitalists on patient outcomes (especially racial), sleep deprivation and fatigue of caregivers, costs of providing this service, and staffing of the labor triage areas in which each patient is evaluated by a qualified clinician before disposition.

DISCLOSURE

The author has no conflicts of interest to disclose.

William F. Rayburn, MD, MBA
Department of Obstetrics and Gynecology
University of New Mexico School of Medicine
Albuquerque, NM 87106, USA

Department of Obstetrics and Gynecology
Medical University of South Carolina
Charleston, SC 29425, USA

E-mail address:
wrayburnmd@gmail.com

Preface

Obstetrics and Gynecologic Hospitalists and Laborists

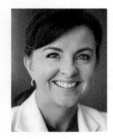 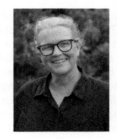

Amy VanBlaricom, MD   Brigid McCue, MD, PhD
Editors

In 2008 the Institute for Healthcare Improvement defined the "Triple Aim" to improve the US health care system by addressing three objectives: improving population health, enhancing patient experience, and reducing per capita cost. In 2017, the Fourth Aim of "improving the work life health of health care providers" was proposed. Most recently, a Fifth Aim acknowledging the impact of health disparities and the need for all providers to strive for health equity, especially among birthing people, was proposed. It has been 9 years since publication of the first issue of *Obstetrics and Gynecology Clinics of North America*, Obstetric and Gynecologist Hospitalists and Laborists. In those years, Ob/Gyn hospitalist work has emerged as a unique practice focus within our field, and Ob/Gyn hospitalists are supporting labor and delivery units across the US from rural hospitals to urban tertiary care centers. The original call to action of the first issue of Obstetric and Gynecologic Hospitalist and Laborist, *Obstetrics and Gynecology Clinics of North America* remains as pressing today: nowhere is the drive and ambition to achieve the (Quintuple) Aim more apparent than in the development and growth of Ob/Gyn hospitalist medicine.

Over the last 30 years, care of hospitalized patients in the United States has been transformed by internal medicine hospitalists, physicians who successfully partner with hospitals to improve care metrics in notable areas, such as prevention of venous thromboembolic events and improvement of care coordination and care transitions.

Ob/Gyn hospitalist medicine initially evolved from similar needs to improve the quality and safety of care for hospitalized women, such as addressing the rising rates of cesarean delivery and leading multidisciplinary teams ready to respond to obstetric emergencies, but also recognized and addressed a critical need for the specialty of Obstetrics and Gynecology to improve the work-life health of physicians in a specialty that, traditionally, has demanded long work hours and time away from home and

Obstet Gynecol Clin N Am 51 (2024) xvii–xix
https://doi.org/10.1016/j.ogc.2024.06.002
0889-8545/24/© 2024 Published by Elsevier Inc.

obgyn.theclinics.com

family. The current crisis of maternal morbidity and mortality, worse among people of color, demands significant improvement in care standardization, patient and provider education, and diversification of our workforce. Obstetric deserts due to shuttered maternity units, and state abortion bans further challenge Ob/Gyn hospitalists, who accept the responsibility to care for the transferred patient, often in dangerous clinical conditions. There is concerted movement toward integrating care models with midwives and other advanced practice nurses to accommodate communities where there are concerns regarding access to care. The field of Ob/Gyn hospitalist medicine strives to positively improve patient outcomes despite each of these evolving hurdles.

This updated issue of *Obstetrics and Gynecology Clinics of North America* provides a summary of topics relevant to Ob/Gyn hospitalist medicine. Multiple experts in the fields of inpatient obstetrics, education of residents and Ob/Gyn hospitalist fellows, patient safety and quality improvement, business development, and diversity, equity, and inclusion efforts have contributed to the issue. Evolving data suggest that Ob/Gyn hospitalists improve quality of care by reducing cesarean delivery rates and improving rates of vaginal birth after cesarean section. Hospitals with Ob/Gyn hospitalist programs demonstrate less maternal morbidity. Ob/Gyn hospitalists are positioned to lead the efforts required by the Joint Commission to reduce harm from obstetric hemorrhage and hypertensive crisis, such as creating policies, initiating drills, and engaging the multidisciplinary team in debriefing. Are there other quality improvement opportunities? For example, can Ob/Gyn hospitalists ensure that the concerns and preferences of people of color and their partners are heard? That black and brown Ob/Gyn residents and fellows are supported and encouraged? That induction of labor is evidence-based, standardized, and tailored to the needs of the individual patient and not to the demands of a physician or health system? Can we design Ob/Gyn hospitalist practices to maximize efficiency, teamwork, and coordination of care while simultaneously balancing these quality and safety improvements and promoting provider longevity and fulfillment?

Twenty-two years have passed since Frigoletto and Greene proposed the practice model of obstetric hospitalists and Louis Weinstein first coined the term "Laborist". The practice of Ob/Gyn hospitalist medicine is well established. This issue of the Ob/Gyn Hospitalist *Obstetrics and Gynecology Clinics of North America* discusses published evidence supporting Ob/Gyn hospitalists successfully achieving the Quintuple Aim to improve population health, enhance patient experience, address issues of cost, improving the work-life health of all Ob/Gyn providers and mitigating the stark impact of health care inequity. Ob/Gyn hospitalists have much more work to do.

DISCLOSURES

The authors have no conflicts of interest to disclose.

Amy VanBlaricom, MD
Obstetrics and Gynecology
OB Hospitalist Group
777 Lowndes Hill Road
Greenville, SC 29607, USA

Brigid McCue, MD, PhD
South Shore University Hospital Northwell
301 East Main Street
Bay Shore, NY 11706, USA

E-mail addresses:
avanblaricom@obhg.com (A. VanBlaricom)
bmccue@northwell.edu (B. McCue)

The Role of the Obstetrics and Gynecology Hospitalist in the Changing Landscape of Obstetrics and Gynecology Practice

Joy Fest, MD, Brigid McCue, MD, PhD*

KEYWORDS

- Ob/Gyn hospitalist • Patient safety • Obstetric care

KEY POINTS

- Obstetrics and gynecology (Ob/Gyn) hospitalist medicine is a growing subspecialty in a dynamic field.
- Emerging evidence shows that Ob/Gyn hospitalists and Ob/Gyn hospitalist programs improve patient safety.
- In an evolving professional landscape, collaboration between Ob/Gyn hospitalists and community Ob/Gyn practitioners is necessary and benefits both clinicians and patients.
- Hospitalists are responsible for maintaining standard of care, implementing evidence-based decisions, promoting a team culture free from implicit or explicit bias, and encouraging structured teaching.
- Ob/Gyn hospitalists must have clinical leadership abilities, knowledge, expertise, and excellent communication skills to support their patients, colleagues, and institutions.

BACKGROUND

The obstetrician and gynecologist (Ob/Gyn) hospitalist continues to be a growing subspecialty of obstetrics and gynecology that is evolving in a dynamic framework. Starting in 2002, leaders in the field recognized the impact of coalescing forces such as the pressure to reduce maternal morbidity and mortality, stagnant reimbursements, the increasing cost of running a private practice, and the demand among practicing Ob/Gyn physicians for an improved work/life balance. Dr Fred Frigoletto, Dr Michael Greene, and Dr Loius Weinstein called for adaptation of the concept of the internal

Department of Obstetrics and Gynecology, South Shore University Hospital, Zucker School of Medicine at Hofstra/Northwell, 39 Montgomery Avenue, Bay Shore, NY 11706, USA
* Corresponding author.
E-mail address: bmccue@northwell.edu

Obstet Gynecol Clin N Am 51 (2024) 437–444
https://doi.org/10.1016/j.ogc.2024.04.001
0889-8545/24/© 2024 Elsevier Inc. All rights reserved.

obgyn.theclinics.com

medicine hospitalist to the field of obstetrics.[1,2] Since then, obstetric units have adopted this model with nearly 40% integrating some form of a hospitalist program.[3] The development and growth of such programs are significantly impacting the changing landscape of the field of obstetrics and gynecology.[3,4]

In 2016, the Society of Ob/Gyn Hospitalists (SOGH; www.societyofobgynhospitalists.com) defined the Ob/Gyn hospitalist as an Ob/Gyn who specializes in the care of hospitalized obstetric and gynecologic patients. The Ob/Gyn hospitalist facilitates care on labor and delivery but may also manage emergent gynecologic surgeries, consults from the antepartum and postpartum units, the emergency department, and inpatient floors. The term *laborist* is frequently used in reference to Ob/Gyn hospitalists but is misleading as it implies an obstetrician/gynecologist who has restricted their professional practice to the care of laboring patients, which is rarely the case. Ob/Gyn hospitalist programs are designed to improve patient safety by minimizing conflicting demands that might delay emergency response and ensuring high-quality patient care.[5]

The scope of care provided by Ob/Gyn hospitalists varies considerably from site to site and can include seeing and evaluating all triage patients in an obstetric emergency department, caring for obstetric patients who lack an assigned practitioner, supporting community Ob/Gyn physicians and nonsurgical obstetric practitioners, such as family medicine physicians and certified nurse midwives, and managing gynecologic emergencies such as ectopic pregnancies. Some Ob/Gyn hospitalists are *maternal fetal medicine (MFM) extenders*, managing complex patients with high-risk pregnancies in close collaboration with the MFM physician who is seeing office patients or consulting from home. Ob/Gyn hospitalists often supervise subspecialty fellows, residents, medical students, and support nursing education, in addition to leading research efforts and quality improvement initiatives. For the purposes of this discussion, the authors use the encompassing term *Ob/Gyn hospitalist*, recognizing that the actual scope of practice may vary.

The concept of the Ob/Gyn hospitalist subspecialist, who has no ambulatory or elective gynecologic surgery practice, with a primary focus of care being patients in the hospital setting is analogous to the role of the internal medicine hospitalist and implies expanded knowledge of hospital systems, use of standardized protocols and procedures, and adherence to quality measures that impact patient safety.[6] In this context, Ob/Gyn hospitalists have an important role to play in the improvement of inpatient care, and provide collaborative support to office-based Ob/Gyn physicians with patients in the hospital setting.[7]

THE CHANGING OBSTETRICIAN AND GYNECOLOGIST LANDSCAPE AND OBSTETRICIAN AND GYNECOLOGIST HOSPITALISTS WITHIN THIS CONTEXT

The field of obstetrics and gynecology is evolving. Such developments can be attributed to both external and internal factors including increased patient acuity and volume, expanding knowledge base and demanding skill sets, insurance reimbursements, rising costs of malpractice insurance, the impact of implicit bias and social determinants of health, desire for an improved work/life balance, demand for work patterns with more flexible or part-time scheduling, and the growth of sub-specializations.[7–9] For example, use of a standardized labor induction protocol has been shown to decrease racial disparities in cesarean delivery rates of Black women (25.7% vs 34.2%; $P = .02$) and neonatal morbidity (2.9% vs 8.9%; $P = .001$) compared with those in an observational group.[10] The increased scope of medical knowledge, technology advancements, and a greater emphasis on physician competencies and certifications have increased extra-clinical demands on obstetricians. For example, patients with a congenital cardiac condition may be managed by a team of perinatologists, cardiologists, perinatal cardiologists, and geneticists in addition to or in place of their primary Ob/Gyn. Redistributing such cases may affect training for residents and opportunities for Ob/Gyn generalists to participate in a more complex case load.[7,11] At the same time, Ob/Gyn physicians who concentrate their practice in a certain area of interest such as management of menopausal symptoms may find it challenging to maintain their clinical and surgical competencies in a wider range of subdisciplines. In addition to the formal Ob/Gyn subspecialties of MFM, Gynecologic Oncology, Urogynecology, and Complex Family Planning, the American Board of Obstetrics and Gynecology (ABOG) now recognizes focused practice certifications for Pediatric and Adolescent Gynecology and Minimally Invasive Gynecologic Surgery, and will consider certification in the near future for Ob/Gyn hospitalists.[8] Within this framework, the prevalence of subspecialized Ob/Gyn physicians is increasing, including more clinicians focusing exclusively on hospital-based obstetrics and gynecology.[7,12] Opportunities for formal subspecialization are increasing, for example, through Ob/Gyn hospitalist fellowship programs, which provide training for the role as an inpatient consultant in acute or emergent cases with the development of relevant clinical skills.[13] The growth of Ob/Gyn hospitalist programs and fellowship training is not only the result of the changing Ob/Gyn landscape but is also contributing to its evolution, with benefits to patients, care teams, and institutions.

OBSTETRICIAN AND GYNECOLOGIST HOSPITALIST PROGRAMS ARE ASSOCIATED WITH IMPROVED CARE

Evidence shows that programs incorporating Ob/Gyn hospitalists decrease the rate of cesarean sections and preterm birth, increase the rate of trial of labor after cesarean delivery and vaginal birth after cesarean, and maintain scores for patient satisfaction.[14–16] Comprehensive obstetric safety initiatives, such as those which included implementation of Ob/Gyn hospitalist programs like at the Yale University and the New York Presbyterian–Weill Cornell Medical Center, achieved substantial reductions in adverse outcomes, malpractice claims, and payouts on malpractice cases.[17,18] Additional components of these initiatives included the use of standardized protocols, obstetric safety nurses, anonymous event reporting, team training, and electronic fetal heart rate monitoring certification—cultural changes facilitated by Ob/Gyn hospitalists. Improvements in staff perceptions of safety as well as a 27% lower odds ratio of cesarean deliveries have been observed after adoption of such initiatives, which included hospitalist models.[6,19] A comparison of safety events at the University of Florida before and after introduction of an Ob/Gyn hospitalist program showed a significant reduction in serious events following implementation.[20] This initial evidence for improved patient safety effected by Ob/Gyn hospitalist practitioners will prove vital as the patient demographic continues to evolve, in particular with the increasing mean age for primigravid women and the corresponding rising rate of associated comorbidities. As work-hour limitations on clinical training may hinder the development of skills and experience, Ob/Gyn hospitalists trained to manage acute obstetric emergencies may become increasingly essential for maintaining patient safety, improving timely management of patients with high-risk pregnancies, and ultimately improving patient outcomes.[13] The potential for optimizing patient care and safety can be attributed to various elements of Ob/Gyn hospitalist programs including those discussed earlier, such as implementing safety protocols and focused training on the management of obstetric emergencies, as well as to the role of hospitalists in leading the coordination of patient-centered care.[8,13,20]

COLLABORATION BETWEEN HOSPITALISTS AND COMMUNITY PRACTITIONERS IS NECESSARY AND BENEFICIAL

Communication and coordination with office-based Ob/Gyn practitioners is essential to the role of Ob/Gyn hospitalists, and teamwork is essential. An Ob/Gyn hospitalist may admit a patient in early labor for the primary Ob/Gyn, cover the epidural, augment with Pitocin, interpret a concerning fetal heart tracing and place an internal lead, while the primary Ob/Gyn finishes their office or surgical day. The primary Ob/Gyn may choose to have dinner with their family and return to take charge of their patient for the delivery or defer to the Ob/Gyn hospitalist. The primary Ob/Gyn might request for the Ob/Gyn hospitalist to assist at cesarean section, and then ask for help managing a postpartum hemorrhage. The Ob/Gyn hospitalist, having managed several postpartum hemorrhages recently, might manage the uterotonic medications, place the uterine tamponade vacuum device and initiate the massive transfusion protocol for the primary obstetric practitioner, then resume care of the patient once she is stabilized, allowing the primary Ob/Gyn to return to other responsibilities. The patient benefits both from the care of her primary Ob/Gyn and their valuable, established relationship, and from the care of the specialized knowledge, expertise, and availability of the Ob/Gyn hospitalist. The primary Ob/Gyn physician benefits from the joy and fulfillment of delivering their longstanding patient but is protected from stress and sleep disruption by the Ob/Gyn hospitalist, improving recruitment and retention of quality practitioners. In this framework, Ob/Gyn hospitalist models allow for more physician control concerning scheduling, greater flexibility, and an overall improvement in work/life balance with higher rates of career satisfaction for both the primary Ob/Gyn and the Ob/Gyn hospitalist.[21] Such coordination between the primary obstetrician and the Ob/Gyn hospitalist improves patient safety through maintaining a collaborative focus on patient-centered care.[20]

While communication and collaboration with office-based practitioners remains essential to the responsibilities of the Ob/Gyn hospitalist, team coordination among hospital staff is also increasingly relevant. Nurse midwives and advanced practice nurses are taking on a vital role in hospital-based obstetric care. Nevertheless, their practice does not extend to the scope of surgical interventions and high-risk perinatal care.[7] Ob/Gyn hospitalists collaborate with all obstetric clinicians and supplement necessary skills in emergent situations, with the ultimate objective of maintaining standard of care.

HOSPITALISTS ARE RESPONSIBLE FOR MAINTAINING STANDARDS AND IMPLEMENTING EVIDENCE-BASED DECISIONS

Emerging evidence has demonstrated that Ob/Gyn hospitalists are a leading force for standardizing obstetric care.[20,22] The Ob/Gyn hospitalist is uniquely positioned to champion cultural changes that lead to improved patient care and decreased adverse outcomes, malpractice claims, and malpractice payouts. The Ob/Gyn hospitalist ensures protocols are followed and quality measures, such as "no elective delivery prior to 39 weeks," are achieved.[18] A cohort study by Srinivas and colleagues confirmed that Ob/Gyn hospitalists could significantly reduce rates of preterm births.[23] The implementation of hospitalist programs with improved, standardized care is furthermore reflected in an associated reduction in the number of malpractice claims per year as well as reduced health care costs.[13,19] Team training and the use of critical communication tools such as briefing, huddles, debriefing and conflict management, championed by the Ob/Gyn hospitalist, spread to the support staff and office-based Ob/Gyn clinicians, and create a culture of safety.[24] As a surgical assist, the Ob/Gyn hospitalist can inform the office-based Ob/Gyn physician of evidence-based findings regarding surgical technique and management, and encourage continuous learning and quality improvement.[25] Within this framework, the potential benefits of implementing comprehensive safety programs and standardized care are a function of Ob/Gyn hospitalists taking on necessary roles as leaders, teachers, and mentors.

HOSPITALISTS ARE LEADERS PROVIDING COMPREHENSIVE SUPPORT

The American College of Obstetricians and Gynecologists /Society for Maternal-Fetal Medicine position paper on levels of maternal care specifies that for level III and above an Ob/Gyn must be on-site at all times.[26] The Ob/Gyn hospitalist in this context is able to provide leadership and expertise for managing transfers to ensure the appropriate care level for each patient, with increased transfer acceptance and increased census in the neonatal intensive care unit. Patients transitioning to the hospital from a planned out-of-hospital birth is an example of a particular challenge regarding trust and acceptance by both the patient and the practitioner.[27] The collaborative leadership role of the Ob/Gyn hospitalist in such situations requires knowledge, strength of character, communication skills, and an ability to connect and empathize with obstetric clinicians and patients. Ob/Gyn hospitalists must use constructive communication to quickly gain the trust of the patient and family, nurses and support staff, primary obstetric clinician, subspecialists, and other hospital staff in the emergency department, operating room, critical care unit, and blood bank, and can lead a team in critical situations.

In addition to developing effective communication skills, core competencies established by the Society of Ob/Gyn Hospitalists encourage Ob/Gyn hospitalists to maintain high-risk, low-volume skills such as forceps, breech delivery of the second twin, and cesarean hysterectomy.[28] Ob/Gyn hospitalists work in defined shifts, limiting the detrimental effect of sleep deprivation and increasing their capacity for then teaching high-risk perinatal care to medical students and residents.[29] They teach by integrating simulations to their labor and delivery team, which has been shown to improve the ability of all practitioners to respond to shoulder dystocia and to increase confidence in responding to maternal cardiac arrest.[30,31] They stay current with the literature and commit to evidence-based practice, implementing safety protocols and clinical pathways, mentoring other physicians to do the same. They maintain ABOG, advanced cardiac life support, neonatal resuscitation program, electronic fetal monitoring, and other relevant certifications, and understand the myriad of quality measures to better advocate for adherence and accurate reporting.

Ob/Gyn hospitalists lead by example. They are uniquely positioned to respond to maternal health disparities, championing efforts to improve diversity, equity, and inclusion on their units and calling attention to acts of implicit and explicit racism that directly impact patients, learners, and colleagues. Mechanisms to reduce disparities such as integrating race, ethnicity, and primary language into quality metrics, maternal mortality and morbidity reviews, and care standardization, and promoting an equitable, just culture, for example, through staff training and patient education are supported by Ob/Gyn hospitalist programs.[32,33] By partnering with community-based doulas and midwives and supporting educational initiatives and curriculum that are diversity, equity, and inclusion focused, Ob/Gyn hospitalists can further directly mitigate racial disparities.[34,35]

As the role of Ob/Gyn hospitalists becomes more defined and integral to the changing Ob/Gyn landscape, Ob/Gyn hospitalist fellowship programs are providing academic opportunities for Ob/Gyn physicians to gain critical experience and develop leadership skills relevant for joining or creating Ob/Gyn hospitalist programs. Ob/

Gyn hospitalist training requires fellows to hone clinical skills for emergent situations and prepares them to be educators with ongoing opportunities to teach residents and medical students through a supervisory role, ultimately improving the quality of teaching and resident satisfaction. Additional responsibilities may include teaching nursing staff, participating in safety committees, involvement in hospital initiatives, and managing the dynamics of academic and community health care systems. Fellowship programs often require research projects and peer review activities. Such structured programs that focus on developing inpatient and emergent obstetric and gynecologic skills as well as clinical leadership will certainly continue to impact and be impacted by the changing landscape of the field.[8,13]

LOOKING AHEAD

The crisis of increasing maternal morbidity in the United States, and especially the inequity in maternal mortality must be addressed.[36] Ob/Gyn hospitalists will meet the growing need for skilled clinicians and leaders in the hospital setting, providing safe and effective, equitable care and comprehensive support to patients, other hospital-based obstetric clinicians, office-based practitioners, academic institutions, and learners. The current demand for Ob/Gyn physician hospitalists is notably high and has led some programs to expand the makeup of the labor and delivery team, including the incorporation of certified nurse midwives and nurse practitioners as Ob/Gyn hospitalists. As the Ob/Gyn landscape continues shift and evolve, the leadership role of Ob/Gyn hospitalists will become further defined and increasingly competitive.[13]

Future goals include establishing and evaluating benchmarks for achieving and maintaining Ob/Gyn hospitalist competencies, including focused practice designation and standardizing fellowship training.[7] As the subspecialty continues to grow, research to further assess Ob/Gyn hospitalist programs will remain crucial. Over the past 10 years, the role of Ob/Gyn hospitalist was defined, programs were established, and the Ob/Gyn hospitalist emerged as the invaluable leader of hospital-based Ob/Gyn care. As safe, evidence-based care continues to evolve in the coming decades, the Ob/Gyn hospitalist will continue to lead their teams and communities in striving for improved care for their patients.

CLINICS CARE POINTS

- Ob/Gyn hospitalist programs improve patient safety.
- Applying evidence-based medicine, maintaining standard of care, promoting diversity, equity, and inclusion initiatives, and teaching among Ob/Gyn hospitalist programs improve clinical outcomes.
- The changing clinical landscape reflects an increased demand for Ob/Gyn hospitalists and the continuously evolving structure of in-patient care for Ob/Gyn patients.

DISCLOSURE

Dr B. McCue reviews for Up to Date.

REFERENCES

1. Frigoletto FD, Greene MF. Is there a sea change ahead for obstetrics and gynecology? Obstet Gynecol 2002;100(6):1342–3.

2. Weinstein L. The laborist: a new focus of practice for the obstetrician. Am J Obstet Gynecol 2003;188(2):310–2.
3. Srinivas SK, Shocksnider J, Caldwell D, et al. Laborist model of care: who is using it? J Matern Fetal Neonatal Med 2012;25(3):257–60.
4. Olson R, Garite TJ, Fishman A, et al. Obstetrician/gynecologist hospitalists: can we improve safety and outcomes for patients and hospitals and improve lifestyle for physicians? Am J Obstet Gynecol 2012;207(2):81–6.
5. What is an Ob/Gyn Hospitalist? In: Society of Ob/Gyn Hospitalists. 2024. Available at: https://societyofobgynhospitalists.org. [Accessed 16 January 2024].
6. Iriye BK, Huang WH, Condon J, et al. Implementation of a laborist program and evaluation of the effect upon cesarean delivery. Am J Obstet Gynecol 2013; 209(3):251.e1–2516.
7. Rayburn W. Who Will Deliver the Babies? Identifying and Addressing Barriers. J Am Board Fam Med 2017;30(4):402–4.
8. Kramer KJ, Rhoads-Baeza ME, Sadek S, et al. Trends and Evolution in Women's Health Workforce in the First Quarter of the 21stCentury. World J Gynecol Womens Health 2022;5(5):622.
9. Royce CS, Morgan HK, Baecher-Lind L, et al. The time is now: addressing implicit bias in obstetrics and gynecology education. Am J Obstet Gynecol 2023;228(4): 369–81.
10. Hamm RF, Srinivas SK, Levine LD. A standardized labor induction protocol: impact on racial disparities in obstetrical outcomes. Am J Obstet Gynecol MFM 2020;2(3):100148.
11. Rayburn WF, Xierali IM. Subspecialization in obstetrics and gynecology: is it affecting the future availability of women's health specialists? Obstet Gynecol Clin N Am 2021;48(4):737–44.
12. Mikhail E. Gynecologic Surgical Training: Current and Future Perspectives. J Gynecol Surg 2022;38(6):372–4.
13. Tatsis V, Butler JR. Implementation of an Academic OB/GYN Hospitalist Fellowship Program: A Sustainable Training Model for Labor and Delivery. J Gynecol Reprod Med 2018;2(1):1–4.
14. Nijagal MA, Kuppermann M, Nakagawa S, et al. Two practice models in one labor and delivery unit: association with cesarean delivery rates [published correction appears in Am J Obstet Gynecol. 2015 Sep;213(3):400]. Am J Obstet Gynecol 2015;212(4):491.e1–4918.
15. Srinivas S, Macheras M, Small D, et al. Does the laborist model improve obstetric outcomes? Am J Obstet Gynecol 2013;208(Suppl 1):S48.
16. Pettker CM, Thung SF, Lipkind HS, et al. A comprehensive obstetric patient safety program reduces liability claims and payments. Am J Obstet Gynecol 2014; 211(4):319–25.
17. Grunebaum A, Chervenak F, Skupski D. Effect of a comprehensive obstetric patient safety program on compensation payments and sentinel events. Am J Obstet Gynecol 2011;204(2):97–105.
18. Clark SL, Frye DR, Meyers JA, et al. Reduction in elective delivery at <39 weeks of gestation: comparative effectiveness of 3 approaches to change and the impact on neonatal intensive care admission and stillbirth. Am J Obstet Gynecol 2010;203(5):449.e1–4496.
19. Pettker CM, Thung SF, Raab CA, et al. A comprehensive obstetrics patient safety program improves safety climate and culture. Am J Obstet Gynecol 2011;204(3): 216.e1–2166.

20. Decesare JZ, Bush SY, Morton AN. Impact of an obstetrical hospitalist program on the safety events in a mid-sized obstetrical unit. J Patient Saf 2020;16(3): e179–81.
21. Funk C, Anderson BL, Schulkin J, et al. Survey of obstetric and gynecologic hospitalists and laborists. Am J Obstet Gynecol 2010;203(2):177.e1–1774.
22. Srinivas SK, Lorch SA. The laborist model of obstetric care: we need more evidence. Am J Obstet Gynecol 2012;207(1):30–5.
23. Srinivas SK, Small DS, Macheras M, et al. Evaluating the impact of the laborist model of obstetric care on maternal and neonatal outcomes. Am J Obstet Gynecol 2016;215(6):770.e1–9.
24. Staines A, Lécureux E, Rubin P, et al. Impact of TeamSTEPPS on patient safety culture in a Swiss maternity ward. Int J Qual Health Care 2020;32(9):618–24.
25. Dahlke JD, Mendez-Figueroa H, Maggio L, et al. The Case for Standardizing Cesarean Delivery Technique: Seeing the Forest for the Trees. Obstet Gynecol 2020; 136(5):972–80.
26. Levels of Maternal Care: Obstetric Care Consensus No, 9 (published correction appears in Obstet Gynecol. 2019 Oct;134(4):883) (published correction appears in Obstet Gynecol. 2023 Apr 1;141(4):864) (published correction appears in Obstet Gynecol. 2023 Apr 1;141(4):865). Obstet Gynecol. 2019;134(2):e41-e55.
27. Snowden JM, Tilden EL, Snyder J, et al. Planned Out-of-Hospital Birth and Birth Outcomes. N Engl J Med 2015;373(27):2642–53.
28. About Society of Ob/Gyn Hospitalists' Core Competencies. 2024. Available at: www.unboundmedicine.com/sogh/view/SOGH-Core-Competencies/2673000/all/. [Accessed 22 January 2024].
29. Clark SL. Sleep deprivation: implications for obstetric practice in the United States. Am J Obstet Gynecol 2009;201(2):136.e1–1364.
30. Draycott TJ, Crofts JF, Ash JP, et al. Improving neonatal outcome through practical shoulder dystocia training. Obstet Gynecol 2008;112(1):14–20.
31. Shields AD, Vidosh J, Thomson BA, et al. Validation of a simulation-based resuscitation curriculum for maternal cardiac arrest. Obstet Gynecol 2023;142(5): 1189–98.
32. Howell EA, Zeitlin J. Quality of care and disparities in obstetrics. Obstet Gynecol Clin N Am 2017;44(1):13–25.
33. Howell EA, Sofaer S, Balbierz A, et al. Distinguishing high-performing from low-performing hospitals for severe maternal morbidity: a focus on quality and equity. Obstet Gynecol 2022;139(6):1061–9.
34. Sobczak A, Taylor L, Solomon S, et al. The effect of doulas on maternal and birth outcomes: a scoping review. Cureus 2023;15(5):e39451.
35. LoGiudice JA. Reducing racial disparities in maternal healthcare: a midwifery focus. SAGE Open Nurs 2022;8. 23779608221138430.
36. Fink DA, Kilday D, Cao Z, et al. Trends in maternal mortality and severe maternal morbidity during delivery-related hospitalizations in the United States, 2008 to 2021. JAMA Netw Open 2023;6(6):e2317641.

Can Obstetrics and Gynecology Hospitalists Reduce Severe Maternal Morbidity?

Joshua S. Brunton, DO, Vanessa E. Torbenson, MD*

KEYWORDS

- Maternal mortality • Severe maternal morbidity • OB/GYN hospitalists
- Safety bundles

KEY POINTS

- Maternal mortality and severe maternal morbidity are on the rise and interventions such as mortality review committees and obstetric safety bundles can be championed by obstetrics and gynecology (OB/GYN) hospitalists as participants and providers of care.
- By providing continuous on-site coverage, OB/GYN hospitalists can reduce response times and mentor other health care providers, including certified nurse midwives, fellows, residents, and medical students, to enhance their skills in obstetric care.
- More study is needed to add to the evidence of the effect of OB/GYN hospitalists in severe maternal morbidity.

MATERNAL MORTALITY

Over the past century, the maternal mortality rate (MMR) has decreased significantly worldwide. In the United States, from 1900 to 2007, MMR decreased from 900 deaths per 100,000 live births to 12.7 deaths per 100,000 live births. The decrease in MMR occurred primarily through general medical advances in care such as antimicrobial therapy, surgical advances, and blood transfusion.[1] Sometime beginning in 2000, MMR began to rise in the United States with an increase from 9.8 per 100,000 live births in 2000 to 21.4 per 100,000 live births in 2014. The increase in MMR is multifactorial, and indeed, one of the factors that may account for up to 79.9% of the rise in MMR from 2000 to 2014 is increased reporting or case capture.[2] Starting in 2003, a question was added to the US standard death certificate inquiring about pregnancy within 42 days of death and within 1 year of the event.

Department of Obstetrics and Gynecology, Mayo Clinic, 200 1st Street Southwest, Rochester, MN 55905, USA
* Corresponding author.
E-mail address: Torbenson.vanessa@mayo.edu

Obstet Gynecol Clin N Am 51 (2024) 445–452
https://doi.org/10.1016/j.ogc.2024.04.002
0889-8545/24/© 2024 Elsevier Inc. All rights reserved.

obgyn.theclinics.com

Incorporation of the pregnancy question was adopted variably in different states through 2014 and this may have accounted for increased ascertainment. One study calculated an adjusted MMR back to 2000 which suggests the MMR in 2000 was closer to 18.8 rather than the previously reported rate of 9.8.[2] While the scale of change of MMR from 2000 to 2014 may be exaggerated due to increased ascertainment, the MMR in the United States continues to rise and represents a significant trend compared to other developed nations.[3]

Coincident to the increase in maternal mortality is the recognition of the disparity in rates between distinct populations: Non-Hispanic Black women experience a rate 3 times that of non-Hispanic white women.[4] This has prompted a call to action to decrease MMR and to address the disparity inherent in obstetric care within the United States.[3]

The components that make up MMR are multifactorial, and any solution will likely include many different building blocks. One group suggests that there should be a systematic creation of maternal mortality reviews . They called for each state to develop a maternal mortality review commitee (MMRC) to review causes of death and identify systemic causes that could be disseminated for quality improvement. Congress enacted the Preventing Maternal Deaths Act in 2018.[5] This law provides federal funding to states for the work done in each state's MMRC. Currently the Centers for Disease Control and Prevention provides funding to 44 states and 2 US territories to support the work of maternal mortality review committees.[6]

Another recommendation to decrease maternal mortality includes the development of safety bundles. Safety bundles are a set of evidence-based practices that when performed can improve patient outcomes.[7] The Alliance for Innovation on maternal health maintains 8 obstetric safety bundles available to individuals and institutions to implement. They include obstetric hemorrhage, severe hypertension in pregnancy, perinatal mental health conditions and sepsis, all relating to diagnoses significantly associated with maternal mortality.[8] Multiple studies have shown an improvement in outcomes, specifically hemorrhage with the institution of safety bundles.[9–11]

SEVERE MATERNAL MORBIDITY

Severe maternal morbidity (SMM) can be defined as unintended outcomes of the process of labor and delivery that result in significant short-term or long-term consequences to a woman's health[12] and can be a proxy to mortality and represent a more frequent outcome that can be studied. SMM is often measured differently in different countries and is sometimes termed a near miss. In one study, SMM occurs approximately 50 times more frequently than maternal mortality.[13] One significant similarity between maternal mortality and SMM are that a significant percentage of cases are preventable.[14,15] SMM then can be used to more frequently track outcomes of quality improvement and reducing SMM or near misses may decrease maternal mortality as a proximate cause.

The major causes of maternal mortality vary by timing in pregnancy and can be viewed in **Fig. 1**.[17] Hemorrhage is a significant cause of maternal mortality at delivery and in the immediate postpartum period and accounts for up to 50% of SMM. This is a significant reason that hospital systems have focused on improving outcomes with hemorrhage and utilizing hemorrhage bundles and best practices. Cardiovascular disease and cardiomyopathy account for a sizable portion of mortality diagnoses after the immediate postpartum period, while hypertensive disorders of pregnancy and infection play significant roles as well. While these medical causes make up a significant portion of maternal mortality and SMM, nonmedical causes, specifically mental

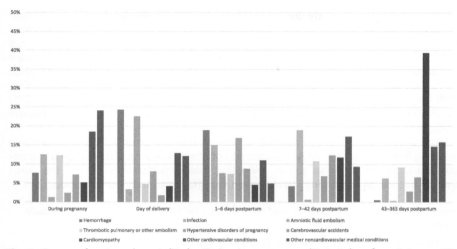

Fig. 1. Causes of maternal mortality by timing in pregnancy. (*Data taken from* Petersen EE, Davis NL, Goodman D, et al. Vital Signs: Pregnancy-Related Deaths, United States, 2011-2015, and Strategies for Prevention, 13 States, 2013-2017. MMWR Morb Mortal Wkly Rep. May 10 2019;68(18):423-429. https://doi.org/10.15585/mmwr.mm6818e1.)

health disorders including overdose, are responsible for up to 50% of pregnancy-associated deaths.

OBSTETRICS AND GYNECOLOGY HOSPITALISTS' ROLE IN MATERNAL MORTALITY RATE AND SEVERE MATERNAL MORBIDITY

Obstetrics and gynecology (OB/GYN) hospitalists, as readily available physicians prepared to respond to emergencies, appear to play a role in decreasing neonatal mortality and morbidity. In a study of data provided by the National Perinatal Information Center/Quality Analytic Services hospitals that compared neonatal outcomes of hospitals with OB/GYN hospitalists and those without, exposed programs had a lower incidence of neonatal preterm delivery.[16] Additionally, a collaborative of 4 hospitals implemented a bundle that included enhanced in-house physician coverage which was associated with a 42% decrease in their adverse outcome index.[18]

Given their ever-ready presence, it has been hypothesized that OB/GYN hospitalists are well poised to aid in the goal of improving maternal outcomes. Clark and colleagues[19] suggested that OB/GYN hospitalists can play a role in decreasing maternal mortality. First through their presence, they can immediately assess patients and diminish delayed diagnosis and treatment which are often responsible for poor outcomes. Secondly, because of their focus on safety initiatives, they are well positioned to improve communication, coordinate care, and provide decisive management to treat patients at risk of morbidity and mortality.[19]

To date, there have been very few studies looking at OB/GYN hospitalists and their role in MMR and SMM. A survey study of American College of Obstetrics & Gynecology (ACOG) and Society for Maternal-Fetal Medicine members reported that[20] 35% of respondents worked in hospitals where OB/GYN hospitalists delivered care.[20] Sixty-nine percent of ACOG respondents felt that the hospitalists were associated with decreased adverse events and 70% felt that they were associated with improved safety/safety culture.[20]

In one observational study, the team administered surveys by telephone and email at hospitals to determine if OB/GYN hospitalists were part of the care team and how they functioned and correlated with hospitals published SMM rates. They found that SMM and the presence of 24/7 coverage increased with the level of neonatal care and delivery volume. They reported that 57% of birthing units had an in-house provider 24/7. They also noted that of hospitals with 24/7 coverage, 54% were staffed by OB/GYN hospitalists while the rest were staff with other providers. Staffing with OB/GYN hospitalists seemed to be associated with a lower SMM for all and low-income mothers.[21]

More outcome studies are needed to assess the role of OB/GYN hospitalists in reducing SMM and MMR. While the initiation of obstetric hospitalist programs is ubiquitous and seems to make sense, relegating their importance to that of the parachute[22] misses an opportunity to improve their effect and their performance.

Important Ways that Obstetrics and Gynecology Hospitalists Can Work to Reduce Specific Maternal Diagnoses

Maternal mental health conditions (including suicide)

Maternal mental health lies at the heart of well-being during the perinatal period, and mental health conditions, particularly postpartum depression (PPD), and anxiety, pose a significant risk to maternal health and contribute to the leading cause of maternal death in the United States. Current estimates suggest an occurrence of approximately 5% to 15% of postpartum women experiencing PPD and around 10% manifesting symptoms of postpartum anxiety.[23,24] However, the intricacies of these conditions warrant a multifactorial approach, as they frequently coexist and may be underdiagnosed. Notably, suicide is a major contributor to maternal mortality during the perinatal period, with perinatal suicide rates in the United States estimated at 1.6 to 4.5 per 100,000 live births.[25]

Addressing these mental health challenges requires a multidisciplinary approach and 3 components set themselves apart: universal screening and early detection, integration of mental health support services, and provider education. Incorporating standardized screening tools, such as the Edinburgh Postnatal Depression Scale or the Patient Health Questionnaire-9, during the prenatal and postpartum visits to improve the identification of signs of anxiety and depression.[25,26] By utilizing these screening tools, health care providers and physicians can target discussions and offer more focused follow-up and referral planning; including and integrating mental health support services into the obstetric care model can allow for timely adjustments to treatment plans, shared decision-making, and improved overall patient care. The final integral aspect to addressing maternal mental health is enhancing health care providers' ability to recognize and manage perinatal anxiety and depression. Developing training programs and communication strategies may increase provider confidence and competence in addressing maternal mental health.

The role of obstetric hospitalists lies within facilitating immediate access to psychiatric consultation and shaping protocols for comprehensive mental health care within the hospital setting. By collaborating with mental health professionals to integrate mental health screenings into routine prenatal and postpartum care, OB/GYN hospitalists can serve as leaders for maternal mental health and aid in facilitating immediate access to psychiatric consultation for high-risk cases. Also, by supporting the development of standardized protocols for the identification and management of perinatal mental health conditions within the hospital setting, OB/GYN hospitalists can ensure that every patient is screened, decreasing bias.

Cardiovascular conditions and hypertensive disorders of pregnancy

Cardiovascular diseases, including hypertensive disorders of pregnancy, represent a significant contributor to maternal morbidity and mortality. To reduce some of the morbidity and mortality related to these cardiovascular conditions, physicians may begin by incorporating comprehensive cardiovascular risks assessments into preconception and prenatal care. By approaching cardiovascular care from a preventative measure standpoint and counseling patients regarding lifestyle modifications, physicians may help reduce adverse outcomes. But importantly, early identification of developing conditions has been shown to reduce the adverse outcomes related to hypertensive disorders of pregnancy.[19] Having a multidisciplinary approach to maternal cardiovascular care is perhaps one of the most crucial aspects to improving outcomes as early involvement of cardiologist, obstetric anesthesiologists, and maternal fetal medicine specialists can improve care coordination and delivery planning for complex cardiovascular patients.

The obstetric hospitalist serves an integral role particularly in the expedient identification and treatment of hypertensive disorders presenting during the intrapartum and immediate postpartum period. As quick medical management and often delivery is the evidence-based treatment for many of these disorders, having a 24/7 hospitalist present on labor and delivery can reduce delays in management.[19,21]

Additionally, as a constant in hospital presence, obstetric hospitalists can provide quick communication with other specialists that may require involvement in complex patient care.

Hemorrhage

Obstetric hemorrhage continues to be a leading contributor to maternal mortality. Many institutions have implemented bundles and protocols to improve outcomes with obstetric hemorrhage. The California Maternal Quality Care Collaborative introduced a safety bundle and showed that collaborative hospitals decreased the rate of SMM from hemorrhage by 20.8% while those in comparison hospitals had a 1.2% reduction.[10] Inherent bundles designed to mitigate the morbidity and mortality of obstetric hemorrhage include active management of the third stage of labor, training programs for the labor and delivery team, and development of standardized protocols for a systematic response to hemorrhages. Obstetric hospitalists can aide in the reduction of hemorrhage, through continuous on-site coverage, enabling prompt recognition and management of severe bleeding, highlighting the importance of immediate availability of obstetric providers. Additionally, the technological space for hemorrhage control has increased in the past several years and obstetric hospitalists who spend a large part of their time on labor and delivery can become experts to deploy this technology.

Infection

Infections during pregnancy and post partum can lead to maternal mortality through systemic complications. Through implementation of infection prevention measures, timely antibiotic administration, and early warning triggers and sepsis bundles, this rising trend of infectious causes of SMM may be able to be reversed. ACOG's safe motherhood initiative endorses several safety bundles including 1 for sepsis. Integral to this bundle is prompt bedside evaluation with worsening status based on vital signs. By serving as a 24/7 presence within the obstetric unit, obstetric hospitalists can provide rapid evaluation of pregnant and postpartum patients aiding in an earlier identification and initiation of treatment for infections. By developing and implementing protocols for workup and expedient initiation of antibiotic therapy, obstetric hospitalists can serve as champions of infection prevention, identification, and early treatment.

Thromboembolism

Pregnancy-related risk of venous thromboembolism (VTE) leading to complications, such as pulmonary embolism and stroke, is another factor contributing to maternal mortality. Some strategies that can potentially reduce the rise in VTE include routine assessment of risk, thromboprophylaxis post partum, and thorough patient education regarding signs and symptoms of VTE. Obstetric hospitalists through their focus on quality and safety can contribute to hospital protocols for prevention, develop educational programs and materials for patients, and actively be involved in risk assessment and early identification of VTE.

General Ways Obstetric Hospitalists Can Reduce Morbidity and Mortality

Medical systems and hospitals might ask, "What is the need for implementing an obstetric hospitalist program?" And the authors present the following as rationale and growing evidence to support the use of obstetric hospitalists.

1. Timely response to complications
   - By providing continuous on-site coverage, obstetric hospitalists are available around the clock, ensuring there is always a skilled professional ready to respond to complications. This immediate availability reduces response times and facilitates timely medical intervention which, as described in the preceding section, is often important for various obstetric complications.
   - As experts in managing obstetric emergencies, such as hemorrhage, infection, preeclampsia, and fetal distress, obstetric hospitalists have a different level of comfort with less commonly seen complications. And by having rapid decision-making and protocolized interventions, obstetric hospitalists can address complications efficiently and effectively.
2. Comprehensive intrapartum and postpartum care:
   - As proficient and competent practitioners in managing labor progression and various delivery scenarios, obstetric hospitalists aim at ensuring safe and efficient deliveries, providing their expertise on labor and delivery units.
   - Obstetric hospitalists do vigilant monitoring during the postpartum course to identify and manage complications promptly being attuned for signs of postpartum hemorrhage, infections, and other post-delivery complications.
3. Care transitions and standardization of care:
   - Through utilization of thorough and routine peer-to-peer sign-out of patients, OB/GYN hospitalists can reduce the loss of patient information and, by following standardized, evidence-based protocols, support institutional and national goals to correct the worsening trends of SMM.
4. Addressing disparities and advocacy:
   - OB/GYN hospitalists can provide tailoring care to address the unique needs of diverse patient populations and aid in developing strategies to reduce health care disparities related to socioeconomic status and ethnicity, which are 2 known contributors to SMM.
   - OB/GYN hospitalists can aid in maintaining involvement in institutional, statewide, and national conversations and committees aimed at reducing maternal morbidity.
5. Capacity building and research contribution:
   - OB/GYN hospitalists can mentor other health care providers, including certified nurse midwives, fellows, residents, and medical students, to enhance their skills

in obstetric care. Through contributing to ongoing professional development programs, obstetric hospitalists can have a wider impact on changing trends in maternal morbidity.

- Through engaging in hospital-based research and actively participating in research initiatives within the hospital setting, obstetric hospitalists have a chance to add to the data on SMM and outcomes of initiatives to help improve these worsening trends. By providing valuable data and insights, obstetric hospitalists can contribute to the improvement of maternal care practices both nationally and internationally.

CLINICS CARE POINTS

- There rise in maternal mortality rate in the US, beginning in 2000, is multifactorial and a portion can be explained by incrase case capture.
- Severe maternal morbidity is a more common occurrence and can be used to monitor outcomes of interventions as a proximate cause of mortality.
- Non-hispanic black women experience a disparity in MMR.
- State MMRC and Safety bundles are interventions intended to decrease MMR and SMM.
- OB/Gyn Hospitalitsts can be readily available to enact safety bundles to improve patient care.
- More research is needed on the impact of OB/Gyn Hospitalists.

DISCLOSURE

The authors report no conflict of interest. The authors received no funding support.

REFERENCES

1. Callaghan WM. Overview of maternal mortality in the United States. Semin Perinatol 2012;36(1):2–6.
2. MacDorman MF, Declercq E, Cabral H, et al. Recent Increases in the U.S. Maternal Mortality Rate: Disentangling Trends From Measurement Issues. Obstet Gynecol 2016;128(3):447–55.
3. Main EK, Menard MK. Maternal mortality: time for national action. Obstet Gynecol 2013;122(4):735–6.
4. MacDorman MF, Declercq E, Thoma ME. Trends in Maternal Mortality by Sociodemographic Characteristics and Cause of Death in 27 States and the District of Columbia. Obstet Gynecol 2017;129(5):811–8.
5. Ahn R, Gonzalez GP, Anderson B, et al. Initiatives to Reduce Maternal Mortality and Severe Maternal Morbidity in the United States : A Narrative Review. Ann Intern Med 2020;173(11 Suppl):S3–10.
6. Prevention CfDCa. Enhancing Reviews and Surveillance to Eliminate Maternal Mortality. 2024. Available at: https://www.cdc.gov/reproductivehealth/maternal-mortality/erase-mm/. [Accessed 13 January 2024].
7. Atallah F, Goffman D. Bundles for Maternal Safety: Promises and Challenges of Bundle Implementation: The Case of Obstetric Hemorrhage. Clin Obstet Gynecol 2019;62(3):539–49.
8. Health AFioM. AIM Patient Safety Bundles. 2024. Available at: https://saferbirth.org/patient-safety-bundles/. [Accessed 13 January 2024].

9. Einerson BD, Miller ES, Grobman WA. Does a postpartum hemorrhage patient safety program result in sustained changes in management and outcomes? Am J Obstet Gynecol 2015;212(2):140–144 e1.

10. Main EK, Cape V, Abreo A, et al. Reduction of severe maternal morbidity from hemorrhage using a state perinatal quality collaborative. Am J Obstet Gynecol 2017;216(3):298 e1–e298 e11.

11. Shields LE, Wiesner S, Fulton J, et al. Comprehensive maternal hemorrhage protocols reduce the use of blood products and improve patient safety. Am J Obstet Gynecol 2015;212(3):272–80.

12. American College of O, Gynecologists, the Society for Maternal-Fetal M, Kilpatrick SK, Ecker JL. Severe maternal morbidity: screening and review. Am J Obstet Gynecol 2016;215(3):B17–22.

13. Grobman WA, Bailit JL, Rice MM, et al. Frequency of and factors associated with severe maternal morbidity. Obstet Gynecol 2014;123(4):804–10.

14. Grechukhina O, Lipkind HS, Lundsberg LS, et al. Severe Maternal Morbidity Review and Preventability Assessment in a Large Academic Center. Obstet Gynecol 2023;141(4):857–60.

15. Collier AY, Molina RL. Maternal Mortality in the United States: Updates on Trends, Causes, and Solutions. NeoReviews 2019;20(10):e561–74.

16. Srinivas SK, Small DS, Macheras M, et al. Evaluating the impact of the laborist model of obstetric care on maternal and neonatal outcomes. Am J Obstet Gynecol 2016;215(6):770.e1–9.

17. Petersen EE, Davis NL, Goodman D, et al. Vital Signs: Pregnancy-Related Deaths, United States, 2011-2015, and Strategies for Prevention, 13 States, 2013-2017. MMWR Morb Mortal Wkly Rep 2019;68(18):423–9.

18. Goffman D, Brodman M, Friedman AJ, et al. Improved obstetric safety through programmatic collaboration. J Healthc Risk Manag 2014;33(3):14–22.

19. Stevens TA, Swaim LS, Clark SL. The Role of Obstetrics/Gynecology Hospitalists in Reducing Maternal Mortality. Obstet Gynecol Clin North Am 2015;42(3):463–75.

20. Levine LD, Schulkin J, Mercer BM, et al. Role of the Hospitalist and Maternal Fetal Medicine Physician in Obstetrical Inpatient Care. Am J Perinatol 2016;33(2):123–9.

21. Torbenson VE, Tatsis V, Bradley SL, et al. Use of Obstetric and Gynecologic Hospitalists Is Associated With Decreased Severe Maternal Morbidity in the United States. J Patient Saf 2023;19(3):202–10.

22. Yeh RW, Valsdottir LR, Yeh MW, et al. Parachute use to prevent death and major trauma when jumping from aircraft: randomized controlled trial. BMJ 2018;363: k5094.

23. Rodriguez AN, Holcomb D, Fleming E, et al. Improving access to perinatal mental health services: the value of on-site resources. Am J Obstet Gynecol MFM 2021; 3(6):100456.

24. Venkatesh KK, Nadel H, Blewett D, et al. Implementation of universal screening for depression during pregnancy: feasibility and impact on obstetric care. Am J Obstet Gynecol 2016;215(4):517 e1–e8.

25. Chin K, Wendt A, Bennett IM, et al. Suicide and Maternal Mortality. Curr Psychiatry Rep 2022;24(4):239–75.

26. Committee opinion no. 453: screening for depression during and after pregnancy. Obstet Gynecol 2010;115(2 Pt 1):394–5.

Obstetrics and Gynecologic Hospitalists and Their Focus
Impact on Safety and Quality Metrics

Alyssa K. Gonzalez, MD[a], Jennifer R. Butler, MD[b],*

KEYWORDS

- Obstetrics and gynecologic hospitalists • Patient safety • Quality metrics
- Nulliparous term singleton vertex (NTSV) • Trial of labor after cesarean (TOLAC)
- Vaginal birth after cesarean (VBAC)

KEY POINTS

- Obstetrics and gynecologic hospitalists improve patient safety by being readily available, being less sleep-deprived, and having a focused practice.
- Obstetrics and gynecologic hospitalists have been associated with decreased length of stay for patients, decreased rates of unnecessary inductions of labor, and decreases in preterm deliveries.
- Obstetrics and gynecologic hospitalists help to reduce cesarean delivery rates.

PATIENT SAFETY

"First do no harm." This is a phrase that has been ingrained in the culture of medicine. Despite this mantra being the guidance that all physicians are imbued with as they begin their practice, patient safety is still an area of medicine that can be improved upon. Humans and systems are not perfect. Therefore, despite the best intentions in caring for patients, some of those patients will be harmed or nearly harmed by the health care system. The field of obstetrics and gynecology is no different. In fact, a labor and delivery floor can at times be the perfect storm that leads to medical errors.

The United States has significantly higher rates of maternal morbidity and mortality than other similarly resourced countries.[1] This concerning trend likely stems from several factors including an aging maternal population and increasing rates of comorbidities in pregnant patients.[2] This creates a need for change in the traditional model of

[a] University of California Irvine, 3800 West Chapman Avenue, Suite 3400, Orange, CA 92868, USA; [b] University of California Irvine, 3800 West Chapman Avenue, Suite 3400, Mail Code: 3200, Orange, CA 92868, USA
* Corresponding author.
E-mail address: butlerjr@hs.uci.edu

Obstet Gynecol Clin N Am 51 (2024) 453–461
https://doi.org/10.1016/j.ogc.2024.05.001
0889-8545/24/© 2024 Elsevier Inc. All rights reserved, including those for text and data mining, AI training, and similar technologies.
obgyn.theclinics.com

labor and delivery. Patients with increasingly complex medical comorbidities create a necessity for a higher level of care.

The traditional model of labor and delivery consists of several private-practice providers caring for patients often remotely. Förster and colleagues conducted a prospective cohort study on one labor and delivery unit to estimate the risk of adverse events. Overall, they found the risk of adverse events to be 2%. In evaluation of the causes of these adverse events, systemic issues such as unavailable providers and nonadherence to protocol were found to be common.[3]

These data show that the traditional structure of labor and delivery in which physicians are remotely monitoring complex clinical scenarios can have negative effects on patient safety. Obstetrics and gynecologic hospitalists are a solution to this issue. Obstetrics and gynecologic hospitalists are physicians that practice primarily inpatient care with limited outpatient/elective surgical responsibilities. Their role is to care for inpatient obstetric and gynecologic patients and manage emergencies.[4]

Torbenson and colleagues conducted an observational study in which they found that severe maternal morbidity was lower in hospitals that had 24/7 labor and delivery coverage by obstetric hospitalists. In contrast to the traditional model of private practice on-call physicians, hospitalist providers are more readily available, better equipped to deal with clinical emergencies due to their focused practice and are less sleep-deprived than their counterparts.[5]

Physician Availability

Patients benefit from having in-house physicians responsible for their care. In fact, the most common area of litigation for malpractice cases is alleged negligence in delayed response of remote physicians and issues of communication between nursing staff and these physicians.[6]

The nature of labor and delivery is highly variable and can change from one second to the next. This coupled with physicians whose attention is being pulled by outpatient visits, scheduled surgeries, and administrative duties leaves room for medical errors that can threaten a patient's safety. Having well trained in-house physicians readily available can fill these gaps and improve the safety and experience of patients.

Obstetrics and gynecologic hospitalists are available for emergent patient needs and can assess fetal heart rate tracings in real time and implement interventions immediately when needed. Additionally, hospitalists can be more easily contacted by bedside nurses in the event of an acute concern such as fetal bradycardia necessitating immediate delivery or evaluation of bleeding concerning for acute placental abruption.

Sleep Deprivation

Another crucial factor to consider in patient safety on labor and delivery is the wakefulness of obstetric providers. Traditionally, obstetricians have cared for patients in labor while also seeing patients in clinic or performing elective surgical procedures. Performing all these functions in addition to often being on call overnight and, therefore, having interrupted sleep can lead to both acute and chronic sleep deprivation. Physicians that are sleep-deprived have impairment in their cognitive and psychomotor skills. Sleep deprivation has been shown to be associated with surgical complications, misinterpretation of data, and impairment in the detection of medical errors.[7]

Sleep-deprived physicians have become the standard for labor and delivery. However, obstetrics and gynecologic hospitalists provide a solution. Hospitalists are not encumbered by outpatient or elective surgical responsibilities, and they typically work shifts and have set hours. Obstetrics and gynecologic hospitalists are more alert and respond to emergencies quickly; they can create a safety net for the labor and delivery unit.

Focused Practice

Obstetrics and gynecologic hospitalists improve patient safety by being well trained and acting as educators and leaders on labor and delivery. Clinical leadership dedicated to improving patient safety has been found to be the most important component in reducing preventable adverse events.[8] Given their constant presence on the labor and delivery unit, obstetrics and gynecologic hospitalists can fill this role in an otherwise disjointed hospital setting. Additionally, because hospitalists are always in-house and have an intimate understanding of the workflow, they can identify areas for improvement and champion safety interventions.

In addition to this, obstetrics and gynecologic hospitalists are well practiced in obstetric emergencies and are well equipped to help respond in these emergencies. Olson and colleagues provide a good example of this in practice. In one community hospital, a new uterine tamponade balloon was introduced. The providers that were able to get training and practice with the balloon were hospitalists, and therefore, they became experts in using this device.[6]

The idea that "practice makes perfect" is truly relevant to clinical providers. One meta-analysis reviewed surgical outcomes from low-volume versus high-volume gynecologic surgeons. The surgeons that operated less were more likely to have intraoperative and postoperative complications.[9] Obstetrics and gynecologic hospitalists can practice their skills daily and, therefore, are more comfortable with procedures like operative vaginal deliveries and can carry them out more safely. This, in comparison to a member of a large private practice that only takes in-patient call on a monthly basis, makes hospitalists safer providers for patients.

An obstetrician's clinical volume has been shown to correlate with the likelihood that a patient's pregnancy will end in cesarean delivery. Clapp and colleagues conducted a retrospective cohort study over 12 years. The primary outcome evaluated was an unscheduled or emergent cesarean delivery that occurred during a patient's labor. Providers were divided into quartiles based on the number of deliveries they performed per year. It was found that patients delivered by physicians below the median of 60 deliveries per year had double the rate of cesarean delivery than their counterparts delivered by higher volume physicians.[10] The focused practice of hospitalists on labor and delivery allows for improvements in the safety of patients and the quality of care they receive.

Clinical Outcomes

Obstetric hospitalists can improve outcomes for laboring patients. Srinivas and colleagues conducted a population cohort study analyzing data from 24 hospitals between 1998 and 2011. The goal of the study was to compare maternal and neonatal outcomes between hospitals with obstetrics and gynecologic hospitalists and hospitals without obstetrics and gynecologic hospitalists. Hospitalist programs were found to be associated with a 15% decrease in the odds of induction of labor and a 17% decrease in odds of preterm birth. No adverse effects were noted as a result of these changes.[11]

Preterm delivery rate is an important target for improvements in patient safety. Preterm delivery is defined as a delivery prior to 37 weeks' gestation. In 2013, 36% of infant deaths occurred because of the sequelae of preterm birth. Most of the morbidity and mortality associated with preterm birth occurs in preterm deliveries less than 32 weeks' gestation.[12] The reductions in preterm delivery that Srinivas and colleagues found were specifically late preterm births. Despite late preterm deliveries being lower risk, they are still associated with the risk of complications such as respiratory distress, jaundice, and greater length of hospital stay. Obstetrics and gynecologic hospitalists reduce rates of unnecessary inductions of labor, specifically those that are late preterm and, therefore, improve outcomes for the newborn.

QUALITY MEASURES

In discussions regarding the safety of obstetric patients, it is important to have clear metrics for tracking the quality of care provided. A quality metric is criterion used to quantify either a specific process or outcome of patient care in comparison to evidence-based data.[13] A variety of quality and outcome measures have been proposed and are being monitored by numerous organizations. Some of these metrics include nulliparous term singleton vertex (NTSV) cesarean delivery rates, episiotomy rates, VBAC rates, early elective delivery rates, and exclusive human milk-feeding rates. In this discussion, we will focus on rates of NTSV cesarean deliveries and rates of vaginal birth after cesarean (VBAC) deliveries.

Cesarean Sections

A significant marker for the quality of care provided by obstetric providers is the rate of cesarean deliveries. Cesarean sections have been associated with increased morbidity and mortality when compared to vaginal deliveries.[14] This is concerning given the increasing rates of cesarean sections. In 2021, 32.1% of all deliveries in the United States were via cesarean section.[15] Rates of NTSV cesarean deliveries have since been established as a marker for quality improvement on labor and delivery. This is the patient population with the lowest risk of cesarean delivery, but the highest consequences for future childbearing.

Implementation of obstetric hospitalist programs has been shown to decrease NTSV cesarean delivery rates when compared to the traditional labor and delivery model. In 2013, Iriye and colleagues conducted a retrospective review of data in a tertiary care hospital between 2006 and 2011. During this time, the hospital's care model changed from the traditional private-practice model to a 24 hour community hospitalist model to finally a full-time hospitalist model. The traditional private-practice model was based on private physicians caring for obstetric patients in the hospital without a rotating call schedule. The community hospitalist model consisted of community obstetricians contracted by the hospital to provide 24 hour coverage for patients that either had no prenatal care or had a provider that did not have privileges in that hospital. Finally, the full-time hospitalist model consisted of obstetricians who were solely employed to provide inpatient care on labor and delivery. The different models of the labor and delivery units are summarized in **Fig. 1**. NTSV cesarean delivery rates were examined during this time, and a 27% odds reduction was noted when comparing the traditional model to the full-time hospitalist model of care. Of note, no significant difference was identified between the traditional model and the community hospitalist model.[16]

In 2015, Rosenstein and colleagues conducted a prospective cohort study between 2005 and 2014 that again showed a reduction in rates of cesarean deliveries with the implementation of an obstetric hospitalist program. This study focused on one hospital in which the labor and delivery model was initially split based on the type of insurance. Privately insured patients were cared for by private-practice physicians that rotated call from either the clinic or home. The publicly insured patients were cared for by midwife/hospitalist coverage in which the midwife provided the majority of

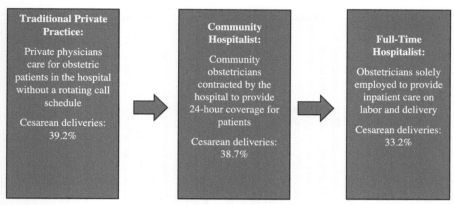

Fig. 1. Models of labor and delivery.

care and had in-house 24 hour hospitalist coverage for back up. The hospital then changed from the traditional private-practice model for the privately insured patients to one with 24 hour midwifery and hospitalist coverage for all patients regardless of insurance type. After this change, a statistically significant decrease in NTSV cesarean delivery rates was noted from 31.7% to 21% for the privately insured patients.[17]

Lastly, the obstetric hospitalist model was once again shown to be associated with decreased NTSV cesarean delivery rates in 2014 when Nijagal and colleagues conducted a retrospective cohort study in a community hospital that included both private-practice and midwife–physician hospitalist practice models. Patients with NTSV pregnancies were significantly more likely to have a cesarean delivery if they were being cared for by physicians utilizing the private-practice model compared with the hospitalist model with an odds ratio of 1.86.[18]

The findings of these studies are summarized in **Table 1**.

Trial of Labor After Cesarean/Vaginal Birth After Cesarean

NTSV cesarean delivery rates are important because in the United States, 90% of patients that require a cesarean delivery with their initial labor will have a repeat cesarean delivery.[19] Along with increasing rates of cesarean deliveries come increasing complications from repeat cesarean sections. Marshall and colleagues conducted a large systematic review and meta-analysis of observational studies regarding repeat cesarean sections. They found that the rate of complications such as hysterectomy, blood transfusions, surgical injury, and adhesive disease all increased with increasing cesarean deliveries. Additionally, they found that the risk of placenta previa and placenta accreta spectrum also increased with increasing cesarean deliveries.[20] To decrease cesarean delivery rates, there has been a push for increased trial of labor after cesarean (TOLAC) attempts. This offers the possibility of a successful VBAC, which has been associated with decreased maternal morbidity, decreased complications in future pregnancies, and decreased rates of cesarean deliveries.[21] Despite the benefits from increased rates of VBAC, TOLAC rates vary dramatically from hospital to hospital. Rosenstein and colleagues in 2013, compared rates of VBACs across California hospitals, which varied from 0% to 44.6%. One of the factors that was found to be associated with increased rates of VBAC included 24 hour obstetric coverage. Additionally, Rosenstein also found an inverse relationship between a hospital's VBAC rate and the primary cesarean rate.[22]

Table 1
Summary of studies evaluating the impact of obstetrics and gynecologic hospitalists on cesarean deliveries

Title and Author	Study Design	Findings
Implementation of a Laborist Program and Evaluation of the Effect Upon Cesarean Delivery Iriye BK, Huang WH, Condon J, et al	Retrospective database evaluation of 3 types of labor and delivery models	• Significant reduction (27.5% reduction) in cesarean delivery seen with the full-time laborist team as compared to the no laborist and community laborist groups • No significant difference between the no laborist and community laborist groups
The Association of Expanded Access to a Collaborative Midwifery and Laborist Model with Cesarean Delivery Rates Rosenstein MG, Nijagal M, Nakagawa S, Gregorich SE, Kuppermann M	Prospective cohort study in a community hospital	• Labor and delivery model changed from private practice to 24 h midwifery and hospitalist coverage. Primary cesarean delivery rate among the privately insured women decreased after the change from 31.7% to 25.0%
Two Practice Models in One Labor and Delivery Unit: Association with Cesarean Delivery Rates Nijagal MA, Kuppermann M, Nakagawa S, Cheng Y	Retrospective cohort study at one community hospital	• Cesarean delivery rates compared between 2 models: private practice and midwifery/hospitalist practice • Women in private-practice model more likely to have cesarean delivery (odds ratio 2.11) • NTSV rate higher in private practice (OR 1.86) • Higher rates of cesarean delivery with history of a previous cesarean (OR 3.19) in the private-practice group

Obstetric hospitalists programs can increase rates of TOLAC/VBAC and reduce the risks of repeat cesareans. By providing around-the-clock coverage on labor and delivery, obstetric hospitalists can provide hospitals and patients with the confidence to safely attempt a TOLAC.

Length of Stay

The term hospitalist was first used in 1996 with the creation of hospital-based internal medicine teams. These programs were initially created to reduce health care costs and length of hospital stay.[6] Obstetrics and gynecologic hospitalists are still working to reduce the length of stay for patients. As discussed, the employment of obstetrics and gynecologic hospitalists has been associated with increased rates of vaginal deliveries and decreased rates of cesarean sections. Therefore, obstetrics and gynecologic hospitalists can decrease hospital length of stay for deliveries. Additionally, hospitalists are less likely to recommend unnecessary inductions of labor and can provide early discharges due to their proximity to the hospital. Both practice patterns can also decrease the overall stay length for patients.

Hospitals can leverage obstetrics and gynecologic hospitalist involvement in quality improvement initiatives leading to awards and accolades such as the US News & World Report Best Hospitals for Maternity Care designation. The purpose of this designation is to allow health care consumers and providers identify hospitals meeting or exceeding perinatal quality benchmarks to better inform decision-making when choosing a hospital. A composite score for maternity care is given based on 8 measures: NTSV cesarean delivery rates, early elective delivery rates, overall unexpected newborn complication rates, routine VBAC rates, exclusive human milk-feeding rates, episiotomy rates, birthing-friendly practice, and transparency on racial/ethnic disparities.[23] Based on current data, the impact of obstetrics and gynecologic hospitalists on other quality measures not discussed in this study is unclear. Given the improvements in the quality of patient care noted with the implementation of hospitalists, more research is needed to determine the impact on other aspects of perinatal quality.

SUMMARY

Obstetrics and gynecologic hospitalists play a pivotal role in the evolution of perinatal care especially as patients and their pregnancies become more medically complex. Hospitalists improve patient safety by providing on-site, reliable, high-quality care. Hospitalists help to reduce the rates of unnecessary cesarean deliveries and increase the rates of vaginal deliveries.

DISCLOSURE

The authors have no commercial or financial conflicts of interest and no funding sources.

REFERENCES

1. Summer SH, Baum CF, Hawkins SS, et al. Severe maternal morbidity in the United States. Econofact; 2023. Available at: https://econofact.org/severe-maternal-morbidity-in-the-united-states. [Accessed 3 January 2024].
2. What factors increase the risk of maternal morbidity and mortality? NICHD - Eunice Kennedy Shriver National Institute of Child Health and Human Development; 2020. Available at: https://www.nichd.nih.gov/health/topics/maternal-morbidity-mortality/conditioninfo/factors. [Accessed 3 January 2024].

3. Forster AJ, Fung I, Caughey S, et al. Adverse Events Detected by Clinical Surveillance on an Obstetric Service. Obstet Gynecol 2006;108(5):1073–83.
4. McCue B, Fagnant R, Townsend A, et al. Definitions of Obstetric and Gynecologic Hospitalists. Obstet Gynecol 2016;127(2):393–7.
5. Torbenson VE, Tatsis V, Bradley SL, et al. Use of Obstetric and Gynecologic Hospitalists is Associated with Decreased Severe Maternal Morbidity in the United States. J Patient Saf 2023;19(3):202–10.
6. Olson R, Garite TJ, Fishman A, et al. Obstetrician/Gynecologist Hospitalists: Can We Improve Safety and Outcomes for Patients and Hospitals and Improve Lifestyle for Physicians? Am J Obstet Gynecol 2012;207(2):81–6.
7. Clark SL. Sleep Deprivation: Implications for Obstetric Practice in the United States. Am J Obstet Gynecol 2009;201(2):136.e1–4.
8. Gluck PA. Patient Safety: Some Progress and Many Challenges. Obstet Gynecol 2012;120(5):1149–59.
9. Mowat A, Maher C, Ballard E. Surgical Outcomes for Low-Volume vs High-Volume Surgeons in Gynecology Surgery: A Systematic Review and Meta-Analysis. Am J Obstet Gynecol 2016;215(1):21–33.
10. Clapp MA, Melamed A, Robinson JN, et al. Obstetrician Volume as a Potentially Modifiable Risk Factor for Cesarean Delivery. Obstet Gynecol 2014;124(4):697–703.
11. Srinivas SK, Small DS, Macheras M, et al. Evaluating the Impact of the Laborist Model of Obstetric Care on Maternal and Neonatal Outcomes. Am J Obstet Gynecol 2016;215(6):770.e1–9.
12. Shapiro-Mendoza CK, Barfield WD, Henderson Z, et al. CDC Grand Rounds: Public Health Strategies to Prevent Preterm Birth. MMWR Morb Mortal Wkly Rep 2016;65(32):826–30.
13. Bailit JL, Gregory KD, Srinivas S, et al. Society for Maternal-Fetal Medicine (SMFM) Special Report: Current Approaches to Measuring Quality of Care in Obstetrics. Am J Obstet Gynecol 2016;215(3):B8–16.
14. Vadnais MA, Hacker MR, Shah NT, et al. Quality Improvement Initiatives Lead to Reduction in Nulliparous Term Singleton Vertex Cesarean Delivery Rate. Joint Comm J Qual Patient Saf 2017;43(2):53–61.
15. Osterman MJK, Hamilton BE, Martin JA, et al. Births: Final Data for 2021. Natl Vital Stat Rep 2023;72(1):1–53.
16. Iriye BK, Huang WH, Condon J, et al. Implementation of a Laborist Program and Evaluation of the Effect Upon Cesarean Delivery. Am J Obstet Gynecol 2013;209(3):251.e1–6.
17. Rosenstein MG, Nijagal M, Nakagawa S, et al. The Association of Expanded Access to a Collaborative Midwifery and Laborist Model with Cesarean Delivery Rates. Obstet Gynecol 2015;126(4):716–23.
18. Nijagal MA, Kuppermann M, Nakagawa S, et al. Two Practice Models in One Labor and Delivery Unit: Association with Cesarean Delivery Rates. Am J Obstet Gynecol 2015;212(4):491.e1–8.
19. Spong CY, Berghella V, Wenstrom KD, et al. Preventing the First Cesarean Delivery: Summary of a Joint Eunice Kennedy Shriver National Institute of Child Health and Human Development, society for Maternal-Fetal Medicine, and American College of Obstetricians and Gynecologists workshop. Obstet Gynecol 2012;120(5):1181–93.
20. Marshall NE, Fu R, Guise JM. Impact of Multiple Cesarean Deliveries on Maternal Morbidity: A Systematic Review. Am J Obstet Gynecol 2011;205(3):262.e1–8.

21. Curtin SC, Gregory KD, Korst LM, et al. Maternal Morbidity for Vaginal and Cesarean Deliveries, According to Previous Cesarean History: New Data from the Birth Certificate, 2013. Natl Vital Stat Rep 2015;64(4):1–13.

22. Rosenstein MG, Kuppermann M, Gregorich SE, et al. Association Between Vaginal Birth after Cesarean Delivery and Primary Cesarean Delivery rates. Obstet Gynecol 2013;122(5):1010–7.

23. FAQ: How and Why We Rank and Rate Hospitals, How and Why We Rank and Rate Hospitals. US News & World Report, Available at: https://health.usnews.com/health-care/best-hospitals/articles/faq-how-and-why-we-rank-and-rate-hospitals (Accessed 6 March 2024).

The Obstetrics and Gynecology Hospitalist
Risk Management Implications

Larry Veltman, MD, CPHRM, DFASHRM[a],*, Victoria N. Ferrentino, Esq[b]

KEYWORDS

- OB hospitalist • OB/Gyn hospitalist • In-house obstetrician • Laborist
- Risk management • Perinatal safety-net • Obstetric emergencies

KEY POINTS

- In-house obstetricians provide a safety-net for management of obstetric emergencies that require expertise and rapid intervention.
- There are substantial data that the presence of obstetrics and gynecology (Ob/Gyn) hospitalists in a perinatal unit improves maternal and newborn outcomes.
- The Ob/Gyn hospitalist enhances risk management activities at multiple levels in the organization.

RISK MANAGEMENT, CLAIMS, GETTING TO HAVARTI

Risk management has evolved as an independent discipline and profession that is based on the classic concepts of loss prevention and loss reduction.
[1] The hospital risk manager may have an independent position or have other combined duties within the patient safety or quality components of the organization, but a significant area of responsibility is the management of medical malpractice claims. According the American Society of Healthcare Risk Management (ASHRM), obstetrics continues to be a leading source of severity of medical malpractice claims.[2] Results of the 2015 Professional Liability Survey conducted by The American College of Obstetricians and Gynecologists (ACOG) (the last such survey conducted) showed that neurologically impaired infant claims were the most common claim against obstetricians (27.4% of 1117 claims); stillbirth or neonatal death was the second most common claim (15% of 1.117 claims). The respondents were asked in the survey to identify other factors that applied to obstetric claims. These included electronic fetal monitoring (22.1%), shoulder dystocia/brachial plexus injury (14.2%), interactions with

[a] 770 Northest Westover Square, Portland, OR 97210, USA; [b] Ferrentino + Brotz, 4488 West Boy Scout Boulevard Suite 400, Tampa, FL 33607, USA
* Corresponding author.
E-mail address: l.veltman@comcast.net

Obstet Gynecol Clin N Am 51 (2024) 463–474
https://doi.org/10.1016/j.ogc.2024.05.002   **obgyn.theclinics.com**
0889-8545/24/© 2024 Elsevier Inc. All rights reserved, including for text and data mining, AI training, and similar technologies.

obstetrics and gynecology (Ob-Gyn) residents (10.6%), and lack of communication between caregivers (10.5%).[3] More recent data from the American Medical Association showed that 62.4% of obstetricians and gynecologists had a liability claim against them at some time during their career.[4]

"Getting to Havarti" is a metaphor proposed by this author to improve safety of obstetric care.[5] The Swiss cheese model of James Reason is an important concept describing how accidents occur in complex organizations.[6] Reason's model suggests that when failures in existing defenses and safeguards line up, the trajectory of a potential accident can penetrate all of the accident protections to cause an injury. The idea of making the holes in the Swiss cheese smaller, that is, "Getting to Havarti" (a Danish cheese with very small holes) is a metaphor for targeting certain areas of a particular perinatal unit to tighten defenses and safeguards so the chance of penetration by an accident's trajectory is reduced and most often deflected. The obstetrician in-house, 24/7, is one strategy that should tighten a perinatal unit's defenses (therefore, reducing the size of the holes) and subsequently reduce the chance for adverse outcomes. In this author's opinion, the safety-net of an in-house obstetrician is one of the best risk management lost prevention strategies available to any perinatal unit, particularly to labor and delivery.

WHAT ARE SOME COMMON OBSTETRIC PRACTICES THAT CAN WEAKEN PERINATAL UNIT DEFENSES? WHAT MAKES THE HOLES IN THE SWISS CHEESE LARGER?

- *The obstetrician may need to be in 3 or 4 places at once.* Because of the demands of an obstetrics and gynecologic practice, a given obstetrician can be scheduled in the operating room, the office, and have patients in labor at 1, and sometimes 2 hospitals all at the same time.
- *High-volume practice.* Booking large number of patients who might be delivering at more than 1 hospital will put stress on the practitioner's ability to see all of these patients in the office as well as attend all of the deliveries.
- *Poor sign out practices.* Multiple providers caring for 1 patient can sometimes result in confusion about changes in the patient's condition or who is in charge of the patient's care at any given time.
- *Inadequate protocols for consultation, referral, or transfer.* This situation can result in confusion and, at times, variation in the timing and the nature of consultation between midwives, family physicians, obstetricians, and perinatologists.
- *Acquiescing to patient requests that are may be unsafe.* There can be the temptation, at times, to yield to pressure from patients, for example, to allow a trial of labor after a previous cesarean (TOLAC) when there may be inadequate "immediately available" personnel or operating room space available during the entire trial of labor.
- *Off-site monitoring of high-risk situations.* The demands of an office practice, the operating room, or the need for sleep can sometimes take the physician away from the patient's bedside during a critical situation.
- *Operation of hierarchy and the lack of teamwork when it comes to safety issues.* Obstetric care has come to be recognized as a team effort and there are occasions when ignoring safety concerns of nurses or house staff can result in failed recognition of a potential problem. Interpretation of fetal heart tracings for instance, benefits from multidisciplinary training, use of standardized definitions, and open communication when conflicts arise.
- *Back up may be inadequate.* Because of the nature of the practice group or the call sharing agreements (or lack of such) within the community, an obstetrician

may find that they are without back up to care for a patient when they are otherwise occupied.

- *Poorly defined roles.* Patient care teams include may nurses, medical students, residents, physicians, midwives, and doulas. It is critical to establish primary, supervisory, and back up roles and to clearly communicate to the patient and their support people the team structure.
- *Failure to recognize the effects of "human factors" on the ability to impair vigilance.* Sometimes physicians find themselves on call for long periods of time. There is ample evidence about the adverse effects of fatigue on the ability to make decisions in health care.[7,8]

THE HOSPITALIST MOVEMENT

In 1996, Wachter and Goldman described a model of care in which hospital-based physicians provided patients' inpatient care in lieu of the patient's primary physician.[9] They termed these physicians, "hospitalists." The hospitalist movement has taken hold and by 1999, 65% of internists had hospitalists in their community and 28% reported using them for inpatient care.[10] In 2003, Louis Weinstein, in an article entitled "The laborist: A new focus of practice for the obstetrician,"[11] advocated for the adoption of the hospitalist model to obstetric care. As of April 2020, the Society of Obstetrician/Gynecologist Hospitalists reported an active membership of almost 1140 individuals.[12]

HOW DOES AN OBSTETRICS AND GYNECOLOGY HOSPITALIST PROGRAM FUNCTION AS A SAFETY-NET FOR A PERINATAL UNIT?

Is the patient's primary physician always available and in-house during labor if an abruption occurs? Who will stand by for a delivery when that primary physician is in route to the hospital for a delivery? Who will manage an unregistered patient who presents to the unit with a prolapsed umbilical cord? Is every patient who comes to triage seen by a physician before discharge? As aptly stated by Clark, and colleagues:

> *Obstetrics today is a team process, requiring the coordinated, integrated involvement of physicians, midwives, nurses, technicians, laboratory support personnel, and the mother. ...Obstetrics in the United States is, (however)...unique in that the traditional captain of the team is often not present during important parts of the labor process.[13]*

Additionally, the human factor of fatigue impacts upon the obstetricians' workload. An individual obstetrician might need to be available for multiple successive nights to manage the labors of multiple patients. With regard to fatigue and its association with a possible deleterious effect on patient safety, a recent ACOG Committee Opinion recommends that "all practitioners ... address fatigue, and efforts should be made to adjust workloads, work hours, and time commitments to avoid fatigue when caring for patients.[14] The Ob/Gyn hospitalist works with the patient's obstetrician to mitigate fatigue.

Does the establishment of in-house coverage with an *Ob/Gyn* hospitalist model actually improve patient safety and reduce claims of malpractice? Clark, and colleagues, in 2008, addressed this issue with the following:

> *A review of almost 200 closed malpractice claims demonstrated that 40% of adverse outcomes related to intrapartum fetal hypoxia, and their associated malpractice claims, may have been avoided had such (in-house) coverage been available.[15]*

Physicians, nurses, and risk managers have all recognized that an in-house Ob/Gyn hospitalist can serve as an important safety-net for the patient care in a variety of ways. These include many of the following:

- Decreasing the chance for precipitous deliveries while the patient's own provider is in transit.
- Rescue of newborn from an abruption or ruptured uterus by performing an emergency cesarean delivery.
- Offering second opinions to both nurses and physicians and mitigating conflict.
- Assisting in surgery with other obstetric emergencies such as shoulder dystocia or postpartum hemorrhage.
- Providing the "immediate availability" of an obstetric surgeon for TOLAC.
- Providing back up for midlevel providers.
- Participating in nursing, medical student, and resident education.
- Assuming leadership roles in drill and simulation design and debriefings.
- Providing emergency call coverage for patients without physicians who present to the emergency department (ED) or to the labor unit.

An example of such an intervention is a case of a primiparous patient laboring at 41 weeks' gestation with reassuring fetal heart tracing demonstrating normal baseline and variability, frequent accelerations, and normal uterine activity pattern. As the labor became more active, at approximately 6 to 7 cm, slightly after midnight the fetal heart tracing demonstrated a prolonged deceleration, which proceeded to a sustained bradycardia with loss of variability. This pattern persisted over the next 10 minutes during transfer of the patient to the operating suite while the attending obstetrician was being called in from home. The Ob/Gyn hospitalist initiated the Cesarean section and delivered a fetus with Apgar scores of 7 at 1 minute and 9 at 5 minutes as the attending was arriving. The arterial cord pH was 7.13, affirming the appropriateness and importance of early intervention and management (Neilson D. Medical Director, Women's Health Services, Legacy Health System, Portland, Oregon, personal communication, 2010).

INTRODUCING THE OBSTETRIC EMERGENCY DEPARTMENT

The obstetric emergency department (OB-ED) is an ED dedicated to the triage and disposition of pregnant patients who present to hospital for various aspects of obstetric care. The OB-ED is often viewed as an extension of the main ED and is, therefore, subject to ED standards of care and accreditation requirements. Algorithms clarify the relationship of the OB-ED and the main ED that defines conditions, gestational ages, and limitations for which patients are evaluated on each respective unit. The location of the OB-ED is most often on the perinatal unit, in proximity to labor and delivery. The key principle of the OB-ED is that every patient is evaluated by a physician or midlevel practitioner before discharge. Some models of the OB-ED have incorporated Certified Nurse Midwives (CNM) into the care model by permanently staffing the OB-ED with a CNM. This allows the OB hospitalist to have more time devoted to patient care and surveillance occurring on the labor and delivery unit.

IS THERE OBJECTIVE EVIDENCE THAT OBSTETRICS AND GYNECOLOGY HOSPITALISTS IMPROVE OUTCOMES AND REDUCE THE CHANCE FOR ADVERSE OUTCOMES?

Studies of maternal and neonatal outcomes that have examined the role of Ob/ Gyn hospitalists as a primary intervention as well as additional studies that have

incorporated Ob/Gyn hospitalists or in-house call as part of an overall perinatal safety program. In 2013, Srinivas, and colleagues, studied 626,772 patients delivered in 24 hospitals. Implementation of laborists resulted in fewer labor inductions, reduced maternal prolonged length of stay, and decreased term neonatal intensive care unit admissions. Additionally, there was a significant reduction in preterm delivery.[16] A theoretic model based on a hospital with 1000 deliveries per month found that the addition of a 24-hour laborist model of coverage would have resulted in improved fetal outcomes. In a population of 100,000 women, 24-hour obstetric coverage resulted in a reduction of 47.1 neonatal deaths per year, 38.4 stillbirths per year, and 24.9 fewer cases of neurologic developmental delay.[17] Barber, and colleagues, showed that a change to a night float (providing in-house physician coverage at night) was associated with a decreased use of induction of labor, an increased likelihood of using oxytocin, and a decreased likeliness to perform manual extraction of the placenta or episiotomy. There were also fewer third and fourth degree lacerations and fewer neonates born with an umbilical artery pH less than 7.10.[18] Gosman, and colleagues, showed that establishment of a rapid response team (of which an in-house maternal-fetal medicine (MFM) specialist or hospitalist was a component) resulted in an increased utilization of this team for various obstetric emergencies.[19] Two studies of comprehensive patient safety initiatives from Yale-New Haven Hospital and New York Weill Cornell Medical Center showed a decrease in overall adverse outcomes. The presence of in house obstetricians was a component of each of these initiatives.[20,21]

Two recent studies validate the value of Ob/Gyn hospitalists with respect to improving perinatal safety. The first, published in 2020, showed a significantly decreased number of safety events after implementation of an Ob/Gyn hospitalist program.[22] The second, published in 2023, showed a significant reduction of severe maternal morbidity associated with the use of Ob/Gyn hospitalists.[23]

All of these studies, as well as wealth of anecdotal experience, point to the risk management benefit to implementing an Ob/Gyn hospitalist program.

THE OBSTETRICS AND GYNECOLOGY HOSPITALIST MOVEMENT AND MODELS OF CARE

An important consideration, which is directly related to patient safety, involves the benefits of the Ob/Gyn hospitalist model in relationship to the work/life stresses and human factors that affect the practice of obstetrics. The practice of obstetrics frequently involves extensive multitasking, working when fatigued, time pressures, sacrificing valued family time, and concern that any error may precipitate litigation. This may lead to an increased risk of burnout which has been shown to increase the chance for errors.[24] Desirable aspects of the Ob/Gyn hospitalist model, as opposed to a more traditional obstetrics/gynecology practice model, include regularly scheduled shifts, more control over work hours, and guaranteed time off.[10]

There are multiple models that have been successful in creating in-house coverage. Each model will have distinct challenges and issues associated with implementation. These issues include the number of full-time equivalents (FTEs) necessary to cover the unit on a 24/7 basis, professional fees or salaries, billing practices, credentialing, professional liability coverage, and the scope of practice of the Ob/Gyn hospitalist. At one end of the spectrum of coverage is to contract with an organization that will provide an entire team of Ob/Gyn hospitalists to cover a given perinatal unit. The other end of the spectrum occurs when the existing community medical staff agrees to provide in-house coverage of the unit on a rotating basis. Coverage by the community obstetricians can be compensated or is sometimes voluntary. There are multiple models that exist along this continuum as alternatives. For example, a hospital may recruit individual Ob/Gyn hospitalists from the community (either locally or nationally) or a hospital could contract with an individual group of obstetricians in the community who agree to provide hospitalist coverage for the unit. There are a number of websites and resources that can be accessed to determine which model is best for a given perinatal unit's volume and make-up.

OVERCOMING CHALLENGES/THE ROLE OF THE RISK MANAGER

The risk manager can help overcome the challenges noted earlier by using patient safety and the safety-net provided by an in-house obstetrician as a central theme. Whether the challenge is the "business case" for safety, patient and practitioner satisfaction, or the establishment of appropriate policies and procedures, the risk manager should take the opportunity to bring the safety aspects of such a program into sharp focus for the entire perinatal and administrative team.

COST

It is clear that any organization considering the addition of Ob/Gyn hospitalists will have to address the costs of such a program. Specifically, when it comes to looking at cost and examining the "business case for safety," the risk manager can work with senior management to gain buy-in regarding safety versus the economic impact of adding an Ob/Gyn hospitalist model. With respect to recouping the costs of such a program, a 2008 study conducted by the Advisory Board estimated that with at a volume of approximately 1000 deliveries per year, a perinatal unit, with active billing procedures, could come close to breaking even for the necessary costs of the additional FTEs.[25] Additionally, the introduction of an OB-ED model may improve the ability to recoup the costs of in-house coverage. It is sometimes difficult to prove prospectively that actual savings will occur with respect to obstetric rescues, decreased liability, and fewer missed deliveries that the Ob/Gyn hospitalist model promises. However, the risk manager, with anecdotes and available data, should play an important role in framing the "business case" in terms of added safety.

PATIENT SATISFACTION

Depending on the Ob/Gyn hospitalist model, patient satisfaction may or may not become an issue. It is common and understandable that patients usually want their physician or midwife to be involved with their delivery. Because care by group practices often divide call, it is common, even without hospitalists, to have physicians or midwives other than the patient's primary caregiver involved with care in labor and delivery. Framing the introduction of the Ob/Gyn hospitalists in terms of patient safety is the best strategy when introducing the Ob/Gyn hospitalist team to the community and individual patients.

PRACTITIONER SATISFACTION

Challenges to the implementation of an Ob/Gyn hospitalist program may occur from practitioners, nursing staff, and administration. Education regarding rescues reminding how an in-house physician can prevent accidents, continued participation in analysis of adverse events and near misses, and ongoing awareness and distribution of literature with regard to Ob/Gyn hospitalists will serve to advance the cause of this safety-net.

Perceived threats that physicians or midwives will be excluded from their own patient's care are common early after initiation of Ob/Gyn hospitalist programs, but these perceptions usually dissipate as the safety elements of the program become real and the true role of the hospitalist become common knowledge. Those who have practiced obstetrics for many years have all missed deliveries, felt the anxiety of having to be in 2 or more places at once, and wished for an immediate assistant in the face of an unexpected emergency. As these situations are addressed and "rescues" occur from having a skilled physician who is always in the hospital, the perceived threats to autonomy are likely to evaporate.

ESTABLISHMENT OF POLICIES AND PROCEDURES SURROUNDING THE OBSTETRICS AND GYNECOLOGY HOSPITALIST MODEL

The leadership of the Perinatal Department (or Division of Obstetrics) should have a multidisciplinary team (to include hospital risk managers) that remains focused on policies, procedures, and operational models to improve patient safety. Clarity about the scope of practice, the limitations of interventions, and communications throughout all levels of the unit should be established with new policies and procedures.

> *A key element for instituting an obstetric… hospitalist program within a facility is the establishment of clear communication methods between…hospitalists and primary health care practitioners. Handoff of patients, updates on progress, and follow-up are all important areas to address because communication gaps are a potential source of patient injury.*[26]

Multiple policies require clear definition. Some of these include issues of safety, issues of billing, and issues of the scope of practice of the Ob/Gyn hospitalist and an effective chain of command that includes important departmental stakeholders should be established to resolve conflicts if and when they arise.

As one looks at the role of the Ob/Gyn hospitalist as an important step along the road to improving patient safety in obstetrics, one should keep in mind the following endorsement from the 2016 Committee Opinion (reaffirmed in 2022) of the American College of Obstetricians and Gynecologists:

> *The American College of Obstetricians and Gynecologists supports the continued development and study of the ob-gyn hospitalist model as one potential approach to improve patient safety and professional satisfaction across delivery settings.*[27]

THE FOLLOWING IS A COMPILATION OF DEFINED DUTIES OF AN OBSTETRICS AND GYNECOLOGY HOSPITALIST DERIVED FROM SEVERAL SAMPLE CONTRACTS

- Maintain high visibility in the department, maintain awareness of clinical activity in the obstetric unit, and have no other clinical or administrative responsibilities during their clinical shift.
- Collaborate with the charge nurse in assuring safe and efficient daily operations via huddles and debriefs, and proactively discuss concerns for patient safety, and function as defined in the chain of command policy for the unit. (The importance of overall unit surveillance cannot be overemphasized. Regular rounding [every 3–4 hours] during each shift with the charge nurse, for example, improves situational awareness and enhances the ability to recognize deteriorating situations in a mother or fetus.)
- Adhere to and support established clinical protocols, identify potentially better practice, and work to implement clinical change and quality initiatives.

- Foster collaborative teamwork among all health care clinicians in the unit, while conducting him or herself in an exemplary professional manner.
- Arrange post discharge follow-up for unassigned patients or unassigned patients seen in triage by the Ob/Gyn hospitalist or CNM.
- Remain aware of labor and delivery patient census and activity throughout the assigned coverage period including:
  ○ Handover at change of shift
  ○ Participation in unit safety huddles
  ○ Periodic assessment of triage patient activity
  ○ Periodic assessment of electronic patient census and fetal tracings on all monitored patients as necessary
- Admit, manage, deliver, and provide inpatient postpartum care for unassigned labor and delivery patients.
- In consultation with MFM, admit, manage, deliver, and provide inpatient postpartum care for unassigned labor and delivery patients or patients transferred to the unit from outside hospitals.
- Provide medical coverage for triage and assure that patients are not discharged from triage without pre-discharge medical review by the attending physician or the Ob/Gyn hospitalist.
- Communicate triage issues to the patient's attending obstetrician by phone as necessary and/or electronically send pertinent information to the attending's office in a timely manner.
- Assist with cesarean deliveries when available.

ED responsibilities for gynecology patients (see discussion as follows on challenges to the unit's safety-net)

- Respond to ED for phone consultation or clinical evaluation for unassigned patients not requiring admission.
- Provide clinical evaluation, initiation of admission history, physical examination, and orders for unassigned patients coming to the ED requiring admission (utilizing a back-up obstetrician for the Ob/Gyn laborist for obstetric duties if necessary).
- Perform minor surgical procedures as obstetric workload permits.

Responsibilities for Departmental Quality and Safety

- Adhere to current practice guidelines, standing orders, and improvement initiatives including those related to infection control, accreditation, and regulatory requirements.
- Advocate for evidence-based safety and consistency in practice.
- Work collaboratively with departmental leadership to identify opportunities for quality, safety or operational improvement through standardization, guideline development, or work process improvement.
- Support the nursing staff as appropriate in review and interpretation of fetal heart tracing and labor progress. This is intended as an educational support role that will help the nurses improve appropriate use of the nomenclature, interpretation skill, and clarity in reporting patient status to the attending physician. Maintain a collegial relationship with staff relative to offering support for clinical decision-making.
- Be familiar with the unusual occurrence report (UOR) process and purpose. Support completion of UORs as mechanisms to identify quality improvement opportunities.

- Lead real time critical incident debriefs on cases in which they are involved.
- Participate in safety rounds and "huddles" with charge nurses, anesthesia clinicians, and staff.
- Be available for obstetric emergencies whether assisting attending or providing direct management in the absence of the attending physician.
- Understand role in chain of command and execute responsibility per chain of command policy.
- Be familiar with essential hospital and obstetric policies, guidelines, and protocols including but not limited to the following:
  - Universal Protocol
  - Medication reconciliation
  - Smoking cessation
  - Drug testing
  - Human immunodeficiency virus testing
  - Hand washing
  - Infection control
  - Electronic fetal monitoring nomenclature
  - Oxytocin administration protocol
  - Massive Fluid Transfusion Protocol
  - Magnesium administration protocol–for tocolysis and pregnancy-induced hypertension if applicable

Additional Responsibilities and Expectations

- Promote patient satisfaction with their experience of care, support a cultural of safety, and meet behavioral expectations to create an environment conducive to mutual respect and learning between physicians and staff. Recognize significance of being the "face of the obstetric unit for patients, attending physicians, and staff." These behaviors are characterized by the following:
  - Collaboration
  - Responsiveness
  - Timeliness
  - Customer service orientation
  - Consensus building
  - Team work
  - Use of situation, background, assessment, recommendation (SBAR) structured communication
  - Pleasant, calm disposition in an environment where uncertainty is present and the ability to multitask is required.
  - Electronic Fetal Monitoring nomenclature and competency training
  - Team training
  - Critical incident debriefing training
  - Simulation training
  - Communication/SBAR
  - Managing difficult people/Critical conversations
  - Review of policies and procedures
  - Competency training for use of electronic medical record

EARLY RESOLUTION, APOLOGY, AND DISCLOSURE

In the last several years, strategies advocating early discussion and resolution, apology, and disclosure associated with unexpected outcomes have become important risk management precepts. Thirty-nine States and the District of Columbia have passed "apology laws" which, to some degree, prohibit expressions of empathy (and in some states, fault) to be admissible in trials[28]; Massachusetts and Oregon have initiated early discussion and resolution legislation.[29,30] Multiple health care systems and professional liability carriers have accumulated data that show the approach to identification of adverse outcomes, early discussions with patients, apology, and disclosure offers significant benefit to the patient, the providers, and to the financial picture of these organizations.[31] The Ob/Gyn hospitalist, through his or her inpatient presence and involvement with patient care, especially in emergencies, often will have objective observations and insight into the issues surrounding an adverse outcome. Through appropriate training, leadership skills, and engagement with other members of the medical staff, the Ob/Gyn hospitalist is in a unique position to participate in any of these early resolution approaches as a result of establishing a strong relationship with the hospital's risk management department.[32]

CHALLENGES TO THE SAFETY-NET

Most OB/GYN hospitalists today are really intended to be OB hospitalists or laborists. Their principal function is to provide in-house coverage of the perinatal unit. However, in some situations, the scope of work outlined in the contract requires the hospitalist to perform gynecology consults in the ED or in the general hospital and also requires them to perform emergency gynecologic surgery, for example, for ruptured ectopic pregnancies or ovarian torsion. This workflow situation takes the hospitalist off of the unit leaving it uncovered for varying lengths of time. This becomes especially important during admission of patients undergoing TOLAC.

Systems need to be implemented to ensure there is the ability to immediately manage a uterine rupture in TOLAC patients when and if the OB hospitalist is called away from the unit. Some units have required that the patient's primary obstetrician or a back-up community physician come to the hospital when the OB hospitalists perform surgery for gynecologic emergencies. Other perinatal units have assigned gynecologic emergency surgery to a community gynecologist on a rotating basis. These approaches all have the function of keeping the OB hospitalist on the unit as much as possible to provide the safety-net for obstetric care that was intended in the first place.

SUMMARY

Most outcomes in obstetrics are favorable. Emergencies, however, do occur and any adverse outcome with respect to a mother or newborn can be devastating to the family, the caregivers, and the institution. Emergency management requires a culture of preparedness and availability of resources. An in-house obstetrician, be it an obstetrician from the community or an independent Ob/Gyn hospitalist fits well with a major risk management precept, that of loss prevention, in the ability to provide a safety-net that provides expertise and eliminates delays in care.

DISCLOSURE

There are no commercial or financial conflicts of interest or funding sources to report.

REFERENCES

1. Orlikoff J, Vanagunas A. Malpractice prevention and liability control for hospitals. Chicago: American Society of Health Systems; 1988.
2. American Society of Healthcare Risk Management. Pearls for obstetrics 2012.

3. ACOG Professional Liability Survey. 2015. Available at: https://protectpatientsnow.org/wp-content/uploads/2016/02/2015PLSurveyNationalSummary11315.pdf.
4. Available at: https://www.ama-assn.org/system/files/policy-research-perspective-medical-liability-claim-frequency.pdf. [Accessed 15 May 2023].
5. Veltman L. Getting To Havarti: Moving Toward Patient Safety In Obstetrics. Obstet Gynecol 2007;110:1146–50.
6. Reason J. Managing the risks of organizational accidents. London: Ashgate Publishing; 1997.
7. Available at: www.rapplaw.com/library/fatigue-and-medical-m.cfm. [Accessed 4 June 2007].
8. Feyer AM. Fatigue: time to recognise and deal with an old problem: It's time to stop treating lack of sleep as a badge of honour.[Editorial]. April 7. Br Med J 2001;322(7290):808–9.
9. Wachter RM, Goldman L. The emerging role of "hospitalists" in the American health care system. N Engl J Med 1996;335:514–7.
10. Auerbach AD, Nelson EA, Lindenauer PK, et al. Physician attitudes toward and prevalence of the hospitalist model of care: results of a national survey. Am J Med 2000;109:648–53.
11. Weinstein L. The laborist: A new focus of practice for the obstetrician. Am J Obstet Gynecol 2003;188:310.
12. Available at: https://societyofobgynhospitalists.org/about-us/. [Accessed 20 May 2023].
13. Clark SL, Belfort MA, Byrum SL, et al. Improved outcomes, fewer cesarean deliveries, and reduced litigation: results of a new paradigm in patient safety. Am J Obstet Gynecol 2008;199:105.e1–7.
14. Committee on Patient Safety and Quality Improvement. Fatigue and patient safety. ACOG Committee Opinion No. 398. American College of Obstetricians and Gynecologists. Obstet Gynecol 2008;111:471.
15. Clark SL, Belfort MA, Dildy GA. Reducing obstetric litigation through alterations in practice patterns experience with 189 closed claims. Am J Obstet Gynecol 2006; 195:S118.
16. Sindhu Srinivas, et al, Does the laborist model improve obstetric outcomes? American Journal of Obstetrics and Gynecology, Supplement, S1-S438, 34th Annual Meeting of the Society for Maternal-Fetal Medicine: The Pregnancy Meeting, February 3-8, 2014, New Orleans, LA, 210:S48.
17. Allen A. The cost effectiveness of 24 hr in-house obstetric coverage American Journal of Obstetrics and Gynecology, Supplement, S1-S438, 34th Annual Meeting of the Society for Maternal-Fetal Medicine: The Pregnancy Meeting, February 3-8, 2014, New Orleans, LA, 210:S48.
18. Barber EL, Eisenberg DL, Grobman WA. Type of Attending Obstetrician Call Schedule and Changes in Labor Management and Outcome. Obstet Gynecol 2011;118:1371–6.
19. Gosman GG, Baldisseri MR, Stein KL, et al. Introduction of an obstetric-specific medical emergency team for obstetric crises: implementation and experience. Am J Obstet Gynecol 2008;198:367.e1–7.
20. Pettker CM, Thung SF, Lipkind HS, et al. A comprehensive obstetric patient safety program reduces liability claims and payments. Am J Obstet Gynecol 2014;211: 319–25.
21. Grunebaum A, Chervenak F, Skupski D. Effect of a comprehensive obstetric patient safety program on compensation payments and sentinel events et al. Am J Obstet Gynecol 2011;204(2):97–105.

22. Decesare JZ, Bush SY, Morton AN. Impact of an Obstetrical Hospitalist Program on the Safety Events in a Mid-Sized Obstetrical Unit. J Patient Saf 2020 Sep; 16(3):e179–81.

23. Torbenson VE, Tatsis V, Bradley SL, et al. Use of Obstetric and Gynecologic Hospitalists Is Associated With Decreased Severe Maternal Morbidity in the United States. J Patient Saf 2023;19(3):202–10.

24. Shanafelt TD, Balch CM, Bechamps G, et al. Burnout and medical errors among American surgeons. Ann Surg 2010;251(6):995–1000.

25. Laborist program breakeven analysis. Washington D.C.: Advisory Board; 2008.

26. The Obstetric–Gynecologic Hospitalist. Committee Opinion No. 459. American College of Obstetricians and Gynecologists. Obstet Gynecol 2010;116:237–9.

27. American College of Obstetricians and Gynecologists' Committee on Patient Safety and Quality Improvement, American College of Obstetricians and Gynecologists' Committee on Obstetric Practice. The obstetric and gynecologic hospitalist. Committee Opinion No. 657. American College of Obstetricians and Gynecologists. Obstet Gynecol 2016;127:e81–5.

28. Ross NE, Newman WJ. The role of apology laws in medical malpractice. J Am Acad Psychiatry Law 2021;49(3):406–14.

29. Available at: http://oregonpatientsafety.org/discussion-resolution/. [Accessed 31 December 2014].

30. Available at: http://www.massmed.org/News-and-Publications/MMS-News-Releases/Landmark-Agreement-Between-Physicians-and-Attorneys-Provides-for-Medical-Liability-Reforms-in-Massachusetts/. [Accessed 31 December 2014].

31. Kachalia A, Kaufman SR, Boothman R, et al. Liability claims and costs before and after implementation of a medical error disclosure program. Ann Intern Med 2010;153:213–21.

32. Hendrich A, McCoy CK, Gale J, et al. Ascension health's demonstration of full disclosure protocol for unexpected events during labor and delivery shows promise. Health Aff 2014;33(1):39–45.

Organizing and Operationalizing an Effective Obstetric and Gynecologic Hospitalist Program

Mark N. Simon, MD, MMM*, Amy VanBlaricom, MD

KEYWORDS

- Obstetric–gynecologic hospitalist • Hospitalist programs • Obstetric emergencies
- Patient safety • Communication

KEY POINTS

- An obstetric/gynecologic (OB) hospitalist program can improve patient safety for obstetric patients on labor and delivery and throughout the hospital.
- The identification and selection of the OB hospitalist team is critical to overall program success.
- Setting up the OB hospitalist program requires setting the appropriate expectations for the OB hospitalists as well as the members of the hospital community.
- Regular feedback on program performance to both the OB hospitalists and the representatives of the hospital allows of continuous quality improvement.

INTRODUCTION

The delivery of obstetric care in the United States consistently attracts much needed attention from policymakers as well as the public. This is largely due to the increase in maternal mortality and morbidity. The Centers for Disease Control and Prevention recently reported that the US maternal mortality rate in 2021 had increased to 32.9 per 100,000 live births.[1] Additionally, the World Health Organization reported that the United States had one of the most significant percentage increases in maternal mortality from 2000 to 2020.[2] These outcomes are driven, in part, by an inability for women to have equitable access to care across the country[3] as well as strain on the obstetric workforce.[4]

One solution to these problems is the implementation of an obstetric and gynecologic hospitalist (Ob/Gyn Hospitalist) program. Ob/Gyn hospitalists have been defined as an obstetrician/gynecologist who specializes in the practice of hospital obstetric

Ob Hospitalist Group, 777 Lowndes Hill Road, Building 1, Greenville, SC 29607, USA
* Corresponding author.
E-mail address: msimon@obhg.com

Obstet Gynecol Clin N Am 51 (2024) 475–484
https://doi.org/10.1016/j.ogc.2024.05.003   **obgyn.theclinics.com**

and gynecologic care.[5] The key to overall success for these programs is to ensure that they have been organized in the most effective way possible. The design must be structured to meet the overarching needs of the program to include

- Delivering quality care for patients to improve clinical outcomes while also reducing liability exposure.
- Allowing the organization to provide obstetric care in the most cost-effective manner possible.
- Addressing the obstetric needs of the community in which the program is located.

We have been involved in the onboarding and management of numerous different obstetrics (OB) hospitalist programs across the United States. While each of these programs has their own unique needs, common themes are evident and this article will strive to help the reader best understand how to begin, operate, and maintain excellent OB hospitalist programs.

DISCUSSION

The first step in operationalizing an excellent OB hospitalist program is to truly understand the needs of the community and hospital in which the program will operate. This requires thoughtful conversations with the local stakeholders including hospital leadership, departmental leadership, nursing representatives, and outpatient obstetric clinicians. Each group may have different definitions of success for the program, and it is critical that the OB hospitalist team understands these and how they all fit together (Table 1). Once the goals for the program have been identified, this should be carried into future touchpoints with the hospital and clinical leadership.

During the program onboarding process, individuals with an operational background should carefully evaluate the current processes and patient flow on labor and delivery. Understanding how patients receive care will ensure that OB hospitalist interactions will be additive and not create inefficiencies. It is also important to confirm that the set-up of the program will meet all regulatory requirements, especially if an obstetric emergency department (OBED) is created. Each state has guidelines that are enforced when designated emergency space is utilized by a hospital. This will include an evaluation of physical layout of the emergency space and its physical relationship with inpatient units. The guidelines have strict requirements to avoid the intermingling of these patient populations. Additionally, patient care rooms in an emergency department

Table 1
OB hospitalist program definitions of success

Potential Questions	Potential Measure of Success
What clinical challenges are currently faced by the department?	Clinical outcome measures focused on the areas of challenge, for example, NTSV rate.
How do community members access obstetric care?	Percentage of delivering patients who initiated prenatal care prior to 15 wk.
What clinicians deliver obstetric care in the community?	Percentage of low-risk deliveries managed by certified nurse midwives/certified midwives.
What is the volume of patients seen in the obstetric emergency department/triage?	Volume of work managed by the OB hospitalist them.
What are the current quality outcomes experienced by patients at this facility?	Change in quality outcomes after implementation of OB Hospitalist program.

have specific size requirements and there will be requirements for the space to have certain equipment available.

INFORMATION TECHNOLOGY AND SYSTEMS INFRASTRUCTURE

The new program will also likely require some changes to the information technology (IT) systems in the hospital. If a new OBED is created, those beds will have to be appropriately designated in the bed management system. Given that the patient care in the OBED will have similarities to both a traditional emergency department and labor and delivery, consideration should be given to the clinical documentation that will be required and how this will work in the hospital's electronic medical record (EMR). Additionally, as an extension of the emergency department, the OBED should track some traditional emergency department metrics such as those associated with patient flow (arrival to room, time to be seen, total time in department).

The hospital and OB hospitalist clinicians will need to be able to bill for the appropriate services provided during a patient's time in the OBED or triage. On the facility fee side, the hospital will need to have systems in place to capture the amount and type of services provided and crosswalk that into the appropriate facility fee level. Implementing this billing structure will require an understanding of how the billing occurs in the emergency department, what tools are used to capture that information, and modifying that or another tool to fit the clinical scenarios most common for obstetric patients. Once the new system process is designed, the staff that will be working in this clinical space will need to be trained on its use. Similarly, the OB hospitalist clinicians will need to be trained to use the appropriate current procedural terminology (CPT) codes for the patients seen. Using the appropriate codes for both the facility and professional services will generate some of the revenue needed to offset the costs of operating a 24/7 facility and having obstetric professionals continually present.

The development or modification of the billing systems will also involve the IT team. The facility charges will need to communicate with the hospital's revenue cycle department while there may need to be the creation of an interface for the OB hospitalist team to create the appropriate professional charges. If the OB hospitalist team utilizes its own system for these charges, it will be important for the hospital to feed the necessary patient demographic data to allow for timely billing. See **Fig. 1** for an overview of the IT interface.

HIRING THE RIGHT OB HOSPITALIST CLINICIANS

Every program requires the hands-on work by the clinical team; therefore, the selection of these team members is critical to program success. Individuals who work in the program must be clinically able to manage the types of patients that they will be expected to encounter. Is this a tertiary care facility or a community hospital? What is the lowest gestational age that is delivered at that hospital? What support services are available? Given these and other factors, what is the comfort level of the candidate to work in that setting? Typically, the strongest OB hospitalist candidates will come from residency programs where they consistently managed a busy, high-acuity labor and delivery unit and worked effectively with other care team members to ensure patient safety. If the candidate comes from a post-residency position, in what type of obstetric environment have they been working? The hiring manager needs to know what type of patients the clinician candidate has cared for in recent years and how that fits with the expected acuity at the hospital.

In addition to clinical skills and acumen, the hiring manager needs to know how this candidate will work as part of the labor and delivery care team. Being an OB hospitalist

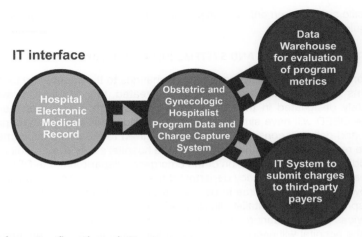

Fig. 1. Information flow through IT systems.

requires collaboration with a variety of health professionals including community midwives, certified midwives, nurses, hospital leaders, and physicians from various departments across the institution. One must be able to navigate whatever political environment exists at that hospital all the while striving to ensure the best possible outcomes for all patients. Communication skills are a key quality that will determine the success of the OB hospitalist.

Patient volumes and acuity can and will vary throughout any given day on labor and delivery. The successful OB hospitalist will be one that is comfortable with uncertainty and can quickly pivot from one patient to another. Again, training in a busy obstetric residency can provide excellent experience for one to refine these skills.

The OB hospitalist in many situations will be expected to serve as a safety champion on labor and delivery. This means that the OB hospitalist should maintain active situational awareness for all patients on the unit and be prepared to intervene or advocate on behalf of the patient. This requires that the OB hospitalist is comfortable engaging with patients they may have had limited interaction with as well as a willingness to challenge the current care plan if it is clear this path could lead to patient harm. These interactions can be challenging as the other physician or midwife may have more years of experience. Additionally, they will likely have a longer standing relationship with the patient. This is why the OB hospitalist should constantly be one to develop relationships with the other clinicians on the unit. By having a trusting relationship with their peers, the OB hospitalist will be in a better position to navigate these difficult conversations when the arise. Regardless, the best OB hospitalist candidates are those that embrace this aspect of the role.

Finally, a successful OB hospitalist will be someone who embraces quality improvement. They identify opportunities for improvement in their own practice or within the hospital processes. They utilize the challenges faced during their daily work to suggest and lead improvement for future patients. This requires an ability to evaluate data, to learn from near misses or undesirable outcomes, and to seek out feedback from all members of the team.

Finding the right people to be a part of any OB hospitalist team puts that program on the road to success. The selection process and criteria need to be robust and relevant to the scope of work that the OB hospitalist will be expected to perform. **Fig. 2** provides an overview of key characteristics of the ideal OB hospitalist candidate.

Key attributes of the ideal OB hospitalist candidate

- Successful track record managing labor and delivery patients (in unit with comparable acuity)
- Highly focused on ensuring patient safety
- Personable and skilled at relationship building
- Licensed to practice medicine in the state of the assigned program
- Excellent communicator
- Team-oriented, service-minded and goal-focused
- Comfortable pivoting from one patient to another
- Embraces quality improvement

Fig. 2. Attributes of OB hospitalist candidates.

Onsite clinical leadership is another important aspect of a successful OB hospitalist program. In addition to the core clinical members of the team, a clinical site director or medical director must be selected. This individual will help to lead the team's clinical quality efforts within the department and interact with local nursing and physician leadership to ensure alignment with the hospital goals. The clinical leader will need to solicit feedback on how individuals are performing and how the team is integrating within the department. They also need to provide feedback to hospital leadership on how the program is being adopted by community physicians and nurses. The clinical site director or medical director role is truly one of ambassador working to balance the needs of the team, the hospital, and the community.

While serving as the ambassador for the program, the clinical site director or medical director also needs to manage the performance of and respond to the needs of their own team members. This requires some managerial skills including serving as the hiring manager, providing regular feedback to their team members, reviewing objective performance measures, and responding to praise and concerns raised by other members of the care team. A successful clinical site director or medical director will have the skills to manage incoming information and pass along to their team. They will also need to regular meetings with their team to share ideas as well as one-on-one interactions.

Ideally, these site directors will provide direct patient care in the hospital as well so that they truly understand the unique dynamics facing the delivery of care. Identification of a clinical leader for the program is another element leading to success (**Fig. 3**).

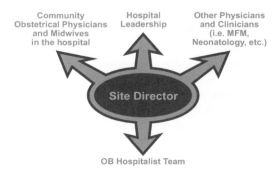

Fig. 3. The role of the site director for the OB hospitalist program.

TRAINING AND ONBOARDING THE OB HOSPITALIST TEAM

Once clinicians have been selected for the OB hospitalist program, they need to be adequately prepared for their first shift. The onboarding experience should include a clear understanding of the objectives of the OB hospitalist program, an overview and introduction to the groups and individual obstetric clinicians with whom the hospitalists will work with, and breadth of clinical conditions that the hospital is capable of managing. The new hospitalists will need to clearly understand hospital processes for managing common obstetric conditions and how emergencies are handled. They also should be familiar with the hospital's protocols for accepting transfers and initiating transfers to other facilities (**Fig. 4**).

New OB hospitalists also must be prepared for their role as clinical obstetric leaders on labor and delivery. This means that they should be up to date on evidence-based care for common obstetric conditions and emergencies such as interpretation of fetal heart rate monitoring, management of shoulder dystocia, management of hypertension in pregnancy, management of obstetric hemorrhage, and standardized communication skills. This education should be required on an ongoing basis so that the team

Hospitalist guidelines provide specific hospital-based details for how OB Hospitalists fit into the hospital clinical structure. Topics include:

Processes

- Communication with community clinicians when patients are seen in the OBED or triage
- Admission of patients to the hospital, particularly when admitted to a community clinician
- How the hospital will manage multiple obstetrical emergencies occurring at the same time
- Scheduling outpatient follow-up after OBED/Triage visits or hospitalization
- Managing laboratory and pathology results, particularly for situations where the results return after patient discharge
- Ensuring that medical record documentation is completed and shared with the patient's primary obstetrical clinician
- Management of inter-hospital transfers
- Scheduling procedures and surgeries
- Ensuring that all deliveries are attended by a licensed independent practitioner

Reminders

- How feedback should be delivered both to the hospitalists and to the unit

Information

- How the chain of command works at the institution
- Other clinical services within the facility such as the NICU, MFM, Anesthesia, Internal Medicine Hospitalist team, Intensivists to name a few.

Fig. 4. Suggested topics for OB hospitalist program guidelines.

stays up to date on the latest scientific advances. **Fig. 5** outlines training requirements for OB hospitalists.

While every program will have its own unique aspects, there will be some core foundational expectations of the work that the OB hospitalist will do and how they will integrate into the existing unit. It is best to spell these expectations out in a formal guideline document. Doing so will provide the new OB hospitalist team with a reference document that can help them be successful during their daily work. At the same time, the document will provide clear communication to the existing nursing and clinical staff on the initial framework for the program. Of course, these can and should be living documents that will change as experience with the program grows. This document should be a collaborative creation of both the OB hospitalist team and the key stakeholders at the hospital so that everyone is operating with a shared vision. Having such a document can prevent conflicts as the program operates and provides a reference to adjudicate any that may arise.

OPTIMIZING THE PROGRAM FOR OPERATIONAL AND CLINICAL SUCCESS

Successful OB hospitalist programs require regular feedback on performance. This means that the program must be designed with the ability to capture data on clinical outcomes as well as operational metrics of program utilization. On the clinical front, the program should monitor outcomes for nationally recognized quality metrics such as NTSV C-section rates, or other low-risk cesarean delivery rates, rates of elective deliveries, episiotomy rates, obstetric harm such as third-degree and fourth-degree lacerations, compliance with hypertension and hemorrhage protocols, and other clinical measures that are relevant to the specific institution. Operational metrics will evaluate the utilization of the program and the capacity for the clinical team to manage additional patients. These should include volumes of patients seen and the

---

Training Requirements for OB Hospitalists

- Interpretation of Fetal Heart Rate Monitoring
- Management of Hypertensive Disorders in Pregnancy
- Management of Obstetrical Hemorrhage
- Management of Sepsis in Pregnancy
- Medical Management of Obstetric and Postpartum Hemorrhage
- Medical Management of Shoulder Dystocia
- Fetal Heart Monitoring
- Use of Standardized Communication Techniques
- Patient Experience of Care
- Understanding Unconscious Bias
- Regulatory Training
  - EMTALA
  - Compliance
- Coding
- Incident Reporting
- Cyber Security

Fig. 5. Suggested training topics for members of the OB hospitalist team.

types of procedures performed, a measure of workload by evaluating the relative work of various procedures, the time spent supporting other physicians or midwives, any support for residency programs to name a few. See **Fig. 6** for recommended quality measures.

The data that are collected should be routinely reported back to the clinicians so that they have an opportunity to see the work that they do and their own clinical outcomes. Additionally, the site director should see the information for their entire team. This allows the leader to identify outliers from whom best practices should be learned or who need additional support in some aspect of their practice. Similar data should be provided to the hospital partner so that there is ongoing dialogue regarding the performance of the program and open communication regarding opportunities for improvement.

No OB hospitalist program can operate successfully in a vacuum. It needs support from individuals with expertise in financial, operational, and quality management. These programs should be managed to improve patient safety and outcomes, minimize financial cost, and maximize operational efficiencies. Financial and operational managers should regularly evaluate the program from these perspectives and offer suggestions to maintain or improve. This includes ensuring that the compensation for the OB hospitalist team remains competitive for the locality in which the program exists. Additionally, the program should be certain to capture all appropriate professional fee revenue from third-party payers. This includes careful evaluation of actual payments as compared to contractual expectations, evaluation of any claim denials, and ensuring that all patient encounters have appropriate claims. The operational experts should also look for opportunities for the program to support additional physicians and midwives in the community. Can the program provide additional coverage for a certain group? Are there Federally Qualified Health Centers that could utilize the services of the OB hospitalists? Are there community midwives who need obstetric consultations? Are there out-of-hospital births that may need support for patients who require transfer to a hospital setting? The operational team can support the clinical team in creating these relationships and facilitating the best collaboration possible.

The inclusion of a supportive quality team will help the clinical team improve their clinical outcomes. Quality experts can evaluate the clinical data for the program and

Obstetric and Gynecologic Hospitalist Program Quality Measures

Quality Measures
Compliance with recognized protocols such as hypertension and hemorrhage management
Vaginal Delivery w. Episiotomy
NTSV w. C-Section
3rd/4th degree laceration (w instrument)
3rd/4th degree laceration (wo. instrument)
OBED patients < 34 weeks EGA w/return < 48 hours

Fig. 6. Suggested measures of clinical success for the OB hospitalist program.

identify areas for improvement. They also partner with the clinicians to implement quality improvement projects with the goal of enhancing patient safety and outcomes. This team should be skilled in analyzing data and providing findings to the clinical team. Additionally, they can coordinate with hospital quality departments to ensure a holistic approach to quality improvement.

Ideally, the clinical team also has more senior clinical leaders upon whom they can rely for clinical support when needed. These regional clinical leaders can provide a broader perspective of successful OB hospitalist programs from their experience with different locations. They are connected with other program support individuals and provide the needed clinical perspective for situations that arise. Having this clinical leader helps to ensure that the program maintains its necessary clinical focus while balancing the financial and operational requirements.

BUILDING RELATIONSHIPS WITH OTHER MEDICAL SPECIALTIES

The clinical team will interact with various other specialties throughout the hospital including maternal–fetal medicine (MFM), neonatology, internal medicine, surgery, intensivists, emergency medicine, and radiology among others. It is imperative that the clinicians build and maintain excellent relationships with these specialties to enhance patient outcomes. Any grievances that arise should be addressed in a timely manner through the leadership of the site director.

The OB hospitalist program should be expected to have a close relationship with MFMs at the hospital. It is important that the program design includes clear expectations on how these two groups will work together. In many cases, the OB hospitalist team will serve as the hands-on clinicians for patients managed by MFM. Having a document that describes the expectations and responsibilities for each group can go a long way in avoiding future conflict.

Similarly, best patient care and outcomes can be promoted when the OB hospitalists and neonatologists have open channels of communication. This will allow for the best information to be provided to patients who might anticipate that their newborn(s) will need care in the neonatal intensive care unit (NICU) while at the same time ensuring that the neonatology team is actively aware of patients at risk of NICU admission.

SUMMARY

Organizing and operationalizing a successful OB hospitalist program requires the dedicated work of many individuals. It is critical to communicate with the hospital to understand how care is currently delivered and their desired goals for the program. The implementation may involve changes to patient flow, development of now policies or procedures, and engagement with IT to modify existing systems and/or connect with new ones. Perhaps the most critical steps for success involve the selection of and preparation of the clinical team. These individuals will be tasked with providing the direct patient care as well as integrating into the political environment at the facility. Finally, there needs to be ongoing measurement of how the program is performing. This involves evaluating the clinical performance of the team as well as the entire labor and delivery unit. Additionally, the program's activity and financial performance needs to be watched. All this information should be communicated transparently with the hospital partner to ensure alignment with their goals and measures of success. Ultimately, successful programs require clear and open communication so that problems, real or perceived, can be addressed quickly. If properly developed and maintained, an OB hospitalist program can provide many years of excellent patient care, improve patient safety and outcomes, all while meeting or exceeding the hospital's goal and measures of success.

CLINICS CARE POINTS

- When developing an OB hospitalist program, all stakeholder should agree on the goals for the program.
- Ensuring that all of the IT systems are properly aligned will lead to a more successful program.
- Choosing the members of OB hospitalist team is a critical step in the development of the program.
- The OB hospitalists and the other members of the clinical team must have a clear understanding of the expectations of the program and its members.
- Developing processes to deliver and receive regular feedback will allow the OB hospitalist program to adapt to the changing needs of the institution.

DISCLOSURE

Both authors are employees of OB Hospitalist Group. There are no other conflicts of interest.

REFERENCES

1. Hoyert DL. Maternal mortality rates in the United States, 2021. NCHS Health E-Stats; 2023.
2. Trends in maternal mortality 2000 to 2020: estimates by WHO, UNICEF, UNFPA, World bank group and UNDESA/population division. Geneva: World Health Organization; 2023. License: CC BY-NC-SA 3.0 IGO.
3. Brigance C, Lucas R, Jones E, et al. Nowhere to Go: Maternity Care Deserts Across the U.S. (Report No.3). March of Dimes. 2022. Available at: https://www.marchofdimes. org/research/maternity-care-deserts-report.aspx.
4. State of the Maternal Health Workforce Brief. Health Resources & Services Administration. 2022. Available at: https://bhw.hrsa.gov/sites/default/files/bureau-health-workforce/data-research/maternal-health-workforce-brief-2022.pdf.
5. McCue B, Fagnant R, Townsend A, et al. Definitions of Obstetric and Gynecologic Hospitalists. Obstet Gynecol 2016;127:393–7.

Triage Versus Obstetric Emergency Department and Main Emergency Department: Best Practices

Amy VanBlaricom, MD*, Mark N. Simon, MD, MMM

KEYWORDS

- Obstetric emergency department • Obstetric emergencies
- Obstetric-gynecologic hospitalist • Patient safety • Obstetric triage

KEY POINTS

- Timely intervention with obstetric emergencies improves outcomes for mother and newborn.
- An obstetric emergency department (OBED) allows for every patient to be seen in a timely fashion by a clinician.
- Understanding state regulations surrounding emergency departments and scope of practice of health care providers are important to implementing an OBED.
- Obstetric-gynecologic hospitalists are uniquely positioned to manage an OBED, however, open communication and trust among community and emergency room clinicians is crucial.

INTRODUCTION

Historically, the evaluation of patients presenting to labor and delivery was via a traditional triage model. In this model, a nurse would initially see and evaluate a patient, determine the urgency of the problem, and reach out by phone to the assigned physician or midwife to request orders for further intervention. The clinician of record would then provide orders over the phone and wait for the nurse to call back with further updates. The clinician might never actually see the patient and would often discharge a patient from triage over the phone. This approach is inconsistent as it requires the nurse to assess and, in some cases, diagnose a patient and present to a physician over the phone. It also requires a nurse to potentially recognize subtle signs of more urgent problems which is outside of their scope of practice. An obstetric triage is not required to have standardized policies and procedures and therefore, care can

Ob Hospitalist Group, 777 Lowndes Hill Road, Building 1, Greenville, SC 29607, USA
* Corresponding author.
E-mail address: avanblaricom@obhg.com

Obstet Gynecol Clin N Am 51 (2024) 485–494
https://doi.org/10.1016/j.ogc.2024.05.005   obgyn.theclinics.com

be inconsistent in evaluating and treating urgent situations promptly, resulting in quality and safety concerns. Obstetric triage is an outpatient service provided in an acute care unit. It is the only place in the hospital where a patient arrives unscheduled for care and ultimately may leave without ever seeing a provider. In addition, because triage is outpatient, the work performed is not adequately attributed to the appropriate unit or department and therefore billing charges and reimbursement on the facility side is significantly less. The word triage defines a process for health care providers to prioritize patients in order of acuity and therefore urgency of need. Unless there is a standardized approach to triage, this process will vary from hospital to hospital and ability to give equitable, timely care will vary based on many local factors.

Contrary to an outpatient triage, an obstetric emergency department (OBED) is an annex of the main emergency department (ED) and therefore, subject to the same policies and procedures as the main ED. EDs have a set of structured triage guidelines that determine which patients need to be seen immediately and which can safely wait while guiding the providers toward appropriate utilization of emergency resources. Patients present unscheduled to an OBED and are seen every time by a licensed clinician. This requires staffing to accommodate the volume of patients arriving through an OBED which, at a busy unit, may require designated clinician staffing. Most pregnant patients present to labor and delivery for an evaluation of labor. In addition to the labor check, assessment of fetal heart rate monitoring is an important component to every labor evaluation. The ability to interpret the evolving fetal heart rate strip in an otherwise routine labor evaluation and intervene where necessary is an important component of the labor work up. Some subsets of those laboring patients may also have developing comorbidities such as preeclampsia requiring additional management. There are also a consequential number of patients presenting specifically for medical comorbidities and urgent problems that require more expertise. When an urgent medical issue is evolving, the time it takes to phone a clinician who is outside the hospital and have them present to the bedside can have catastrophic implications to both the mother and the fetus. Thus, having a licensed clinician see and evaluate every unscheduled patient on a unit in a timely fashion allows for such evaluation and when needed, delivers urgent or emergent care.

ADVANTAGES TO AN OBSTETRIC EMERGENCY DEPARTMENT

There are 2 types of EDs. A type A ED is one that provides emergency services 24 hours per day, 7 days per week and is beholden to the Emergency Medical Treatment and Labor Act (EMTALA) regulations. A type B ED is beholden to the EMTALA but does not meet the requirement of 24/7 care. An example of a type B ED is a free-standing emergency room that is not open overnight. As labor and delivery is a 24/7 operation, an OBED would typically be a type A ED.[1] A compliant type A OBED offers notable advantages in terms of patient safety and satisfaction as every patient is seen by a licensed obstetric provider. The required time of arrival to being seen in the OBED is the same as the main ED. Therefore, the time from arrival to being seen in an OBED is significantly shorter than an outpatient triage which allows for necessary emergency interventions based on acuity. This not only impacts patient safety, but also patient satisfaction as the patient also has an opportunity to discuss their care directly with the provider and have their questions answered. Delay in diagnosis and delay in care are between 23% and 63% of medical malpractice claims.[2] Given the significant improvement in time to assess and treat in the OBED, it stands to reason that bad outcomes stemming from such delays would be mitigated significantly and along with it, malpractice claims. For all of these reasons, standardized, timely, expert emergency care that is offered to all presenting patients every time, is considered best practice.

In terms of finances, as an OBED is an annex of the main ED, facility fee charges are consistent with that of the main ED and higher than an outpatient triage, where there are no professional fees as the patients are not seen by a clinician. Other advantages to an OBED are outlined in **Fig. 1**.

CONSIDERATIONS WITH IMPLEMENTATION

Successful implementation of an OBED requires collaboration with multiple departments and a high degree of communication with the main ED staff. For example, a determination of gestational age cut off to be seen in the OBED must be determined.[3] Many choose 16 or 20 weeks and above to be seen in the OBED. However, if the main ED is very busy and staffing on labor and delivery allows, some may decide to see patients at lower gestational ages in the OBED, such as 12 weeks. There is also the question of postpartum patients and where they will be seen. Given a high percentage of patients with severe maternal morbidity present postpartum, it makes sense in some situations to have those patients be seen directly in the OBED.[3,4] Once it is determined which patients will be seen in the main ED and which ones will be seen in the OBED, it is particularly important to make sure there are streamlined processes for evaluation by an obstetric provider for those patients that remain in the main ED but ultimately need consultation with obstetrics. There will be occurrences where a patient presents above the gestational age cutoff to the main ED, or presents with a non-obstetric concern that makes more sense to be evaluated in the main ED such as severe asthma, lacerations, or fractures not related to abdominal trauma and others. Open communication with main ED personnel when this occurs will maintain appropriate level of care and efficiency of time. Other departments important to the successful OBED implementation are listed in **Fig. 2**.

Determination of which patients are seen in main ED versus OBED needs to be done in conjunction with staffing determinations. An OBED requires designated, appropriately credentialed nursing, available clinicians for patient care and a high degree of communication with community providers as patient expectations will need to be managed as well. Physicians in the community will need to message their patients that an OBED means a copay when not admitted and that they should present only for concerns that require evaluation on labor and delivery. This may require

OBED Advantages

- A "specialty" emergency department- e.g. PEDS, ORTHO, GERIATRIC, NEURO etc.
- All patients seen by a licensed clinician (MD,DO, CNM etc.)
- Improved door to doc disposition time
- Improved patient satisfaction
- Improved quality/safety and decreased med/mal exposure
- Decreased volume stress on main emergency department
- Improved facility and professional fee reimbursement
- Creates a revenue/cost center

Fig. 1. OBED advantages.

Departments Involved in a Successful
OBED Implementation

- Main emergency department (gestational age limit, postpartum patients)
- Labor and delivery unit
- Information technology/Health information technology
- Finance/Revenue integrity
- Compliance/Risk
- Facility management
- Department of Health rules and regulations
- Community practices

Fig. 2. Departments involved in a successful OBED implementation.

modifications to office phone triage and staffing to accommodate those patients who can be seen in the office. The clinician in the hospital evaluating patients in the OBED must establish a bridge of trust with the community provider and acceptable communication about the status of their patients to ensure that information and need for follow-up is made clear.

A successful OBED implementation requires compliance with the same rules as the main ED. This means, OBED designation as a unit in the electronic medical record, a dedicated space on or near labor and delivery with appropriate signage, access to a restroom and waiting area, a dedicated nurse, dedicated clinician (physician, midwife, or nurse practitioner depending on the scope of practice in your state) and the ability to bill appropriate facility and professional charges through a designated cost/revenue center. Other commonalities between an OBED and main ED are listed in **Fig. 3**.

A NOTE ABOUT THE EMERGENCY MEDICAL TREATMENT AND LABOR ACT

The EMTALA requires any hospital with a designated ED to provide a medical screening examination to any patient presenting with an emergency medical condition, including labor.[5] It also prohibits hospitals with an ED from refusing a medical screening examination to patients who present requesting one. The need for the medical screening examination is determined by the presenting patient requesting it, not by the clinician providing it. This means, any patient who presents to a hospital with a request for emergency care must at minimum, receive a medical screening examination by an appropriate provider. Ultimately, the patient should be either managed by that provider or stabilized and transferred to another facility if the initial facility does not have the appropriate capability to treat the patient. A "qualified clinician" to perform the medical screening examination is determined by hospital policy and typically outlined in the bylaws. The list of qualified individuals could include a certified nurse midwife, physician, or nurse, depending on the situation and scope of practice delineation. Ultimately this means that as a designated annex to the main ED, every patient that presents to the OBED must receive a medical screening examination by a qualified provider. As obstetric hospitalists are qualified providers (including certified nurse midwives), they play an important role in maintaining compliance with the EMTALA.

TEAM AND EXPERTISE

Consideration of staffing, training, and credentials is of paramount importance in successful OBED implementation. Nurses who will be working in the OBED will require

> ### The OBED functions as an extension of the main emergency department with the same rules, regulations, policies and procedures.
>
> - Emergency Medical Treatment and Labor Act (EMTALA)
> - Billing & coding (Acuity scoring)
> - Compliance
> - Regulatory
> - State regulations
> - Physical **specifications**
> - Policy and procedures
> - Registration
> - Training & education
> - Reporting (internal & external)
> - Transfers (In and out)
> - Clinician electronic medical record documentation

Fig. 3. The OBED functions as an extension of the main ED with the same rules, regulations, policies, and procedures.

additional education on policies, procedures, the EMTALA, and definition of medical screening examination among other things. There are rules about who can be assigned to the OBED based on this education and credentials so it is important to work with the nursing staff to designate who on any given shift, will be assigned to the OBED and what that means to the rest of staffing on the labor floor. Determination on whether and in what situations each level of staff can perform a medical screening examination is also important and would be dictated by hospital policy. Of note, as the OBED is a designated annex to the main ED, it benefits from more urgent throughput of requests for radiology, laboratory tests and other diagnostic and therapeutic tests and interventions under the label of "emergency department."

Additionally, a standardized triage tool to quickly assess acuity upon arrival has been shown to benefit patients through timely care in addressing urgent and emergent needs. These tools allow for those patients with the most urgent needs to be prioritized to maximize timely treatment and efficiency of care. There are several such tools being used today, most of which were not developed specifically for the concerns of pregnant patients. One validated obstetric triage assessment tool is the maternal-fetal triage index created by the Association of Women's Health Obstetric and Neonatal Nurses. This tool is widely available and can serve as the tool for a unit or as a template for a unit specific tool adjusted for unique hospital circumstances. For the maternal fetal triage index file, visit www.awhonn.org/ and select education tools.[6]

There needs to be a designated provider to see every patient in the OBED in a timely fashion. Depending on the anticipated OBED volume, this may mean an additional provider to cover the rest of the labor deck. As obstetric hospitalists are in house 24/7, and are experts in the diagnosis and management of obstetric emergencies, they are perfectly positioned to manage the OBED alongside designated nursing staff.[7] Obstetric hospitalists are adept in standardized diagnostic algorithms, checklists and protocols which allow for standardized, timely, expert care. Obstetric hospitalists are also

Sample algorithm: Patient presents to maternity

Patient w/OB symptoms

- Patient brought to OBED. OB unit secretary arrives the patient. Labor & delivery admitting completes registration. If patient is experiencing acute medical symptoms call for main ED response.

Patient assessed in OBED by OB hospitalist or patient's OB/GYN within 30 minutes. If OB/GYN unavailable within 30 minutes, OB hospitalist assesses patient.

- Patient admitted
- RN transfers out of OBED to inpatient bed

- No need for admission
- Patient discharged with follow-up instructions

Patient with non-OB symptoms

- After assessment, main ED/OB triage form determines if patient goes to OB RN calls main ED triage RN
- Determination made whether patient can be safely transferred to main ED versus calling rapid response
- Patient admitted to main ED by main ED admitting

Patient in main ED
Main ED RN calls OB charge RN to assess baby (Doppler/Non Stress Test) if deemed necessary by physician

Reactive Non Stress Test
- Main ED care continue to either admit or discharge
- OB RN gives OB instructions for home (AVS)

Non-Reactive Non Stress Test
- Main ED MD assesses patient for treatment and care and decides patient disposition
- OB/GYN provider consulted for next steps

Fig. 4. Sample algorithm: Patient presents to maternity.

trained in availing themselves to hospital resources to support barriers to communication such as interpreter services, social services, and culturally sensitive care. Additionally, as the obstetric hospitalist is present to care for all patients, agnostic to their insurance status, ability to pay or other demographics, they mitigate the impact these demographics have on care and begin to address inequities in care based on demographics. Obstetric hospitalists are also ideal safety champions on the labor unit, taking ownership of drills and simulations of obstetric emergencies and ensuring all staff are adept at emergency protocols and that the entire labor unit team is high functioning, efficient and effective. Having appropriate policies, procedures, clinical protocols, safety bundles, and checklists that are built into the electronic medical record and posted throughout the OBED is best practice as they contribute to timely, expert, standardized care that will benefit patients. See algorithm **Fig. 4**.

PHYSICAL SPACE

When determining whether the physical space on labor and delivery can appropriately accommodate an OBED, there are multiple elements to consider. Every state will have a unique conversion process and it is important to understand the regulatory requirements in your state. Licensing of the beds under an emergency room license is a universal need. However, in most cases, a new ED license is not needed, as the OBED would be added to the existing ED license. There are additional requirements regarding signage

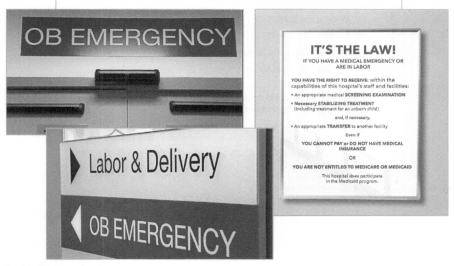

Communication

How will the OBED be communicated by outpatient practices and onsite?

- Ensure appropriate signage identifying the OBED and EMTALA verbiage is posted in easily viewable locations such as waiting rooms, registrations and entry to the units

- Acknowledge and communicate that copays/co-insurances/deductables are not eliminated if the community provider completes the OBED exam instead of the OBHG physician.

Fig. 5. Communication.

to designate the OBED as an emergency room (**Fig. 5**), appropriate space for the waiting area, layout that does not involve walking past inpatient beds to arrive at registration, and appropriate technical set up of the space in terms of security and medical gases in the OBED bed areas. The local department of health may require an inspection as well as the fire marshal. In some cases, if the layout of the labor and delivery unit does not meet the state requirements, construction may need to occur requiring inspection as well. Prior to an inspection it is a good idea to walk the unit and run several patient presentation scenarios to work through patient and staff flow. See **Fig. 6**.

INFORMATION TECHNOLOGY AND HEALTH INFORMATION TECHNOLOGY

There are several information technology (IT) components to an OBED that need to be considered, streamlined and tested for flow prior to OBED go live. These include patient registration, unique department designation on the electronic medical record (EMR), a unique charge master and virtual beds to name a few. A conversation with the hospital EMR representative may help to configure appropriate templates and order sets as well (**Fig. 7**). Having all these components in place and tested via multiple

OBED Physical Space and Team

- Coordination of personnel
  - Director of Women's Services, facilities, emergency department, labor and delivery, information technology, health information technology, **finance,** compliance/risk
- Appropriate **signage/wayfinding**
- Demonstrate separate and **identifiable** resources from the labor and delivery unit
- Dedicated OBED beds (as an emergency bed) necessary gas lines, space for gurneys etc.
- Restroom access
- Does not cross over inpatient thresholds
- Waiting room access
- Nurse workstation
- Registers patients as emergency department patients
- Available with physician coverage 24 hours a day/7 days a week
- Demonstrates and documents collaboration as one emergency department
  - Operates under a set of policies and procedures consistent with the main emergency department
  - Adopts similar acuity scoring and pricing methodology

Fig. 6. OBED physical space and team.

OBED Information Technology Components

- Registration
- Clinician documentation
- Patient disposition
- Ability to track CMS metrics
- Tracking board
- Communication with main ED
- Charge master
- Virtual beds
- May require conversations with hospital EMR
- Consider ED module vs. labor and delivery
- Creating new beds affects many depts such as laboratory, radiology, pharmacy

Fig. 7. OBED information technology components.

Elements of a Successful OBED Site Survey

- Ensure that emergency department and labor and delivery have physically walked the floorplan together and run various presentation scenarios to ensure patient flow works
- Have binder prepared based on what local office is asking to review
  - Policies and procedures
  - Map/floorplan showing physical relationship from main emergency department to OBED
  - Staff training materials: How was the staff oriented? Sign offs from the staff from education and in-service sign in sheets
  - Planned quality indicators ex. Door to doc times
  - Supplies and equipment list stored in OBED
  - Test patient in the EMR

Fig. 8. Elements of a successful OBED site survey.

simulated dry runs prior to a state survey will significantly improve the likelihood of a successful survey. See **Fig. 8**. Working through alternative scenarios for patient and nursing flow is also important. What if a patient who should have come to OBED presents to main ED? What if a main ED patient presents to the OBED? Considering the physical space, urgency of patient status, and capacity of OBED will all be important in these uncommon but real scenarios. Ultimately having multiple simulated patients run through registration and the EMR combined with a physical walk through of the OBED space to determine efficiency of flow will allow any changes and-or process improvements prior to taking the OBED live.

SUMMARY

Historically, unscheduled patients were evaluated on labor and delivery via a traditional triage model that involved a nurse evaluating the patient and corresponding with the responsible clinician over the phone. This method was not standardized and made labor and delivery the only location in the hospital where patients would present unscheduled and not be seen by a qualified clinician on a consistent basis. It has been shown that having a provider in the hospital available to see and evaluate every patient in a timely fashion improves care and patient satisfaction. A model is considered best practice when it requires standardized, consistent, timely evaluation and care by a qualified clinician every time. The OBED allows for these elements and confirms the ability to bill and be reimbursed in alignment with emergency room charges which are more appropriate for the resource allocation required for this kind of care. Obstetric hospitalists are present in the hospital, trained and experienced in management of obstetric emergencies and therefore uniquely poised to provide this care in collaboration with frequent communication with main emergency room staff. The Society for OB/GYN Hospitalists has taken this one step further, developing a core competency delineation around the role an obstetric hospitalist plays in the OBED/triage.[8] There are many elements to be considered when implementing an obstetric ED. With forward planning and collaboration with stakeholders in the emergency, IT, nursing and physical plant departments, a successful conversion from triage to OBED can occur.

CLINICS CARE POINTS

- Unscheduled visits to an OBED as opposed to a triage allow timely evaluation by a qualified provider of care every time.
- Coordination with the main emergency department allows every patient to have appropriate, timely evaluation by a qualified specialty provider to their presenting complaint.
- An OBGYN hospitalist run OBED, allows compliance with EMTALA.

DISCLOSURE

Both authors are employees of Ob Hospitalist Group. There are no other conflicts of interest.

REFERENCES

1. https://www.cms.gov/medicare/medicare-fee-for-service-payment/hospitaloutpati entpps/downloads/opps_qanda.pdf
2. Wallace E, Lowry J, Smith SM, Fahey T. The epidemiology of malpractice claims in primary care: a systematic review. BMJ Open 2013;3(6):e002929. June 18.
3. ACOG Committee Opinion. Hospital-Based Triage of Obstetric Patients. Number 667. July 2016 reaffirmed 2023. ACOG website.
4. Srinivas SK. Potential impact of obstetrics and gynecology hospitalists on safety of obstetric care. Obstet Gynecol Clin N Am 2015;42:487–91.
5. EMTALA. https://www.cms.gov/medicare/provider-enrollment-and-certification/cer tificationandcomplianc/downloads/emtala.pdf.
6. Ruhl C, Scheich B, Onokpise B, et al. Content validity testing of the maternal fetal triage index. J Obstet Gynecol Neonatal Nurs 2015;44(6):701–9.
7. ACOG Committee Opinion. The Obstetric and Gynecologic Hospitalist. Number 657. February 2016 reaffirmed 2022. ACOG website.
8. SOGH Website Ob/Gyn Hospitalists' Core Competencies. Obstetric Triage Emergency Department. SOGH website.

OBGYN Hospitalist Fellowships

An Update on Fellowship Training in the United States

Anthony Grandelis, MD[a],*, Vasiliki Tatsis, MD, MS, MBA[b]

KEYWORDS

- Hospitalist • Academic • Fellowship • Education • Labor and delivery
- Patient safety

KEY POINTS

- Obstetrics & Gynecology (OBGYN) hospitalist fellowships were developed to train the future leaders of hospital medicine and inpatient clinician experts.
- OBGYN hospitalist fellowships can help recent residency graduates improve their confidence and competency in managing high-risk and emergent cases in OBGYN, as well as learn essential hospitalist skills not typically taught in residency.
- As fellowship programs continue to expand across the country, particular importance will need to be paid to recruitment and improving awareness regarding the importance of these programs.

THE OBGYN HOSPITALIST MOVEMENT

Developed just over 20 years ago, the OBGYN hospitalist model of care has seen exponential growth and is now implemented by many hospitals across the country. Inspired by the internal medicine hospitalist programs, the concept of a laborist was introduced in 2002 to decrease burnout and improve physician well-being, while concurrently improving patient safety[1] amidst increasing rates of maternal and infant morbidity and mortality. As this model gained traction, the Society of OBGYN Hospitalists (SOGH) was formed in 2010 with a mission to improve outcomes for hospitalized OBGYN patients. Today, the role of an OBGYN hospitalist includes providing care for patients in labor and delivery (L&D), the antepartum unit, the postpartum unit, the general emergency department, and the obstetric emergency department.[2]

[a] Department of Obstetrics and Gynecology, Columbia University, 622 West 168th Street, New York, NY 10032, USA; [b] Department of Obstetrics, Gynecology, and Reproductive Sciences, University of CA, San Francisco, 490 Illinois Street, 9301, San Francisco, CA 94143, USA
* Corresponding author.
E-mail address: Ajg2302@cumc.columbia.edu

Obstet Gynecol Clin N Am 51 (2024) 495–501
https://doi.org/10.1016/j.ogc.2024.05.009   **obgyn.theclinics.com**

Additional responsibilities of OBGYN hospitalists may include serving as inpatient Maternal Fetal Medicine (MFM) extenders; playing an active role in quality and safety; educating residents, fellows, and medical students; providing L&D support for private obstetricians; and leading simulations for obstetric emergencies.[2,3]

For many years, the proposed benefits of OBGYN hospitalists remained purely theoretical. However, literature has emerged in the last decade that overwhelmingly supports the continued growth of this model. Specifically, it has been shown that OBGYN hospitalists can improve the primary cesarean delivery rate (as well as nulliparous term singleton vertex cesarean delivery rate),[4–6] increase the likelihood of successful vaginal birth after cesarean, decrease rates of preterm births,[7] reduce the number of malpractice claims, lessen the incidence of critical safety events,[8,9] enhance resident and medical student education,[10] improve rates of severe maternal morbidity,[11] and close the gap in racial disparities in care.[12] As a result, it is anticipated that demand for OBGYN hospitalists will continue to increase.

THE HISTORY OF OBGYN HOSPITALIST FELLOWSHIPS

Despite a need for more OBGYN hospitalists, there has historically been a shortage of qualified physicians to fill these roles.[13] Based on a 2010 survey, OBGYN hospitalists at the time were more likely to be physicians with more than 15 years of experience.[14] As they approached retirement, employers began looking to recruit the next generation of OBGYN hospitalists. Unfortunately, recent OBGYN residency graduates were rarely choosing this as a career path, in part due to unforeseen consequences of duty hour restrictions, decreased resident autonomy, and a worsening medico-legal environment.[13,15] Since the early 2000s, there has been a steady decline in the national average of many core OBGYN procedures performed by ACGME resident graduates.[3] Specifically for obstetrics, there has been a declining rate in overall vaginal deliveries as well as operative deliveries, with forceps-assisted deliveries seeing a greater decline than vacuum-assisted deliveries. Competence in breech vaginal deliveries has also decreased, with only 11% of graduating residents planning to offer vaginal breech deliveries to their patients.[15]

Furthermore, a survey completed by OBGYN fellowship directors (female pelvic medicine and reconstructive surgery, gynecologic oncology, maternal–fetal medicine, and reproductive endocrinology-infertility) regarding preparedness for advanced clinical training revealed that graduating residents are perceived to have deficits in professionalism, independent practice, psychomotor skills, clinical evaluation, and academic scholarship. Interestingly, this survey revealed that residents are well prepared from an obstetrics standpoint but lack necessary gynecologic skills, including competency with abdominal hysterectomies. Finally, this report showed low performance ratings of new fellows in recognition and management of critically ill patients.[16]

Due to the aforementioned concerns, employers may be hesitant to hire recent graduates for OBGYN hospitalist positions, and they often require prospective hires to have several years of experience after residency training.[13] In response, an OBGYN hospitalist fellowship was proposed as a safe "bridge" to enhance skills and confidence of recent OBGYN graduates interested in a career as an OBGYN hospitalist.[3] In addition, fellowship training could allow for development of important nonclinical skills, such as quality improvement, simulation development and implementation, and leadership.

As a result, the first OBGYN hospitalist fellowship was developed at NYU Langone Hospital in Long Island, New York, and the first fellow was enrolled in 2013.[13] Since that time, the number of OBGYN hospitalist fellowships programs has grown, and today, the SOGH recognizes 10 non-ACGME-accredited programs (**Table 1**). Following is a discussion regarding the landscape of OBGYN hospitalist fellowships across the country. Utilizing information from program-specific Web sites (see **Table 1**), as well as expert opinion from past and present fellowship directors (see acknowledgments), the remainder of this article will attempt to summarize key differences and similarities across programs, as well as review important considerations for those hoping to start a fellowship at their own institution.

DIFFERENCES AND SIMILARITIES ACROSS OBGYN HOSPITALIST FELLOWSHIPS

Currently, the biggest differences between programs are the length of training (1 year vs 2 year programs) and clinical setting (academic vs community programs). With regard to length of training, 5 programs currently offer 2 year programs (see **Table 1**) and cite several reasons for the extra year. Some fellowship leaders believe that achieving clinical competency requires 2 full years of additional training. This is of particular importance for some clinical skills, such as forceps deliveries or peripartum hysterectomies. Additionally, an extra year allows for more time to develop meaningful scholarly projects and perhaps obtain an advanced degree, such as a master's degree in Public Health, Business Administration, or Applied Science in Patient Safety and Quality.

This emphasis on nonclinical training is what sets fellowships apart from other OBGYN hospitalist apprenticeships offered by OB hospitalist employment agencies. Unfortunately, the cost of providing advanced degrees as part of fellowship training may not be feasible within a program's budget. Additionally, recruiting for a 2 year program means deferring 2 years of attending-level salary, which may not be appealing to some applicants. Thus, the optimal duration of OBGYN hospitalist fellowship training is still up for consideration given the aforementioned factors.

Another difference between fellowship programs is clinical setting. In academic programs, benefits include access to a breadth of clinical research and quality improvement support. Additionally, these programs may offer the benefit of training at a referral center, which allows for more exposure to high-risk pregnancies, placenta accreta centers of excellence, and learners at all levels of training. In community programs, fellows may have the opportunity to train without resident physicians, which may allow for more primary hands-on experience. Community programs can also provide the unique experience of teaching L&D nurses, which can increase patient safety and nursing satisfaction. Given that both academic and community programs have unique advantages, some fellowships have designed their program to include training at both types of institutions.

Although differences do exist, by and large the objectives and clinical duties are similar across the 10 fellowships. Ultimately, the goal is to create the future leaders in OBGYN hospitalist medicine, which includes training fellows who are clinically proficient in providing evidence-based care to hospitalized OBGYN patients, including management of high-acuity and complex cases. Thus, clinical training is focused on L&D, OB triage, antepartum care, ultrasonography, inpatient gynecology, and emergency room gynecology consultations and surgical management. In addition, given the secondary goal of training fellows who will pursue hospital leadership roles, there is a universal component of quality improvement and patient safety training, with most programs requiring a scholarly project within this domain.

CONSIDERATIONS FOR STARTING AN OBGYN HOSPITALIST FELLOWSHIP

When preparing to start an OBGYN hospitalist fellowship, there are many important considerations. First, it is critical to gain departmental support, including buy-in from

Table 1
Current OBGYN hospitalist fellowships recognized by the Society of OBGYN Hospitalists

Program	Location	Number of y of Training	Web Site
Ascension Saint Thomas Hospital Midtown	Nashville, TN	2	https://comnashville.uthsc.edu/content/ob-gyn-hospitalist-fellowship/
Northwell Health South Shore University	Bay Shore, NY	1	https://professionals.northwell.edu/continuing-professional-education/fellowship-obgyn-hospitalist-program-south-shore
NYU Langone Hospital—Long Island	Mineola, NY	1	https://medli.nyu.edu/departments-divisions/obstetrics-gynecology/education/obstetrics-gynecology-hospitalist-fellowship
Mayo Clinic	Rochester, MN	2	https://college.mayo.edu/academics/residencies-and-fellowships/obstetrics-hospitalist-fellowship-minnesota/
University of California, Irvine	Irvine, CA	2	https://www.obgyn.uci.edu/hospitalist-fellowship.asp
Baylor College of Medicine, Texas Children's Hospital	Houston, TX	1	https://www.bcm.edu/departments/obstetrics-and-gynecology/education/fellowships/hospitalist-fellowship
University of Texas, Houston—Memorial Herman	Houston, TX	2	https://med.uth.edu/obgyn/education/fellowships/mcgovern-medical-school-uthealth-ob-gyn-hospitalist-fellowship-training-program
University of California, San Francisco—Kaiser	San Francisco, CA	1	https://obgyn.ucsf.edu/fellowship-training-programs/ucsf-kaiser-obgyn-hospitalist-fellowship
University of Colorado, Anschutz Medical Center	Aurora, CO	1	https://medschool.cuanschutz.edu/ob-gyn/fellowships/ob-gyn-hospitalist-fellowship
Cleveland Clinic	Cleveland, OH	2	https://my.clevelandclinic.org/departments/obgyn-womens-health/medical-professionals/education-programs/obgyn-hospitalist-fellowship

https://societyofobgynhospitalists.org/portfolio/fellowships/.

key stakeholders in divisions that will be involved in training the fellow. Examples include MFM, General OBGYN, Gynecologic Oncology, Minimally Invasive Gynecology, and nursing leadership on L&D. With regard to securing funding, most programs have been able to hire the fellow as a clinical instructor since the fellowship is not ACGME accredited. This strategy is financially attractive to hospital leadership because the fellow can bill for patient care while maintaining a PGY5-6 salary.

Another daunting task can be curriculum development, especially considering the lack of standardization at this time. Most fellowship programs have utilized the SOGH Core Competencies for OBGYN hospitalists as a model for curriculum design (https://www.unboundmedicine.com/sogh), and some programs recommend concurrently designing the fellowship based on ACGME accreditation requirements for other fellowship programs (https://www.acgme.org/globalassets/pfassets/programrequire ments/cprfellowship_2022v3.pdf). This will allow for an easier transition if OBGYN hospitalist fellowships become ACGME accredited. In an effort to standardize fellowship training, the SOGH Fellowship Committee is currently working on a standardized curriculum as well as basic minimum criteria for fellowship program implementation.

One important aspect of curriculum design includes a plan for graduated autonomy. In other words, how will the program ensure adequate supervision of the fellow during the beginning of their training, and how will this transition to greater autonomy as the fellowship progresses. Some programs have moved to a 2 physician coverage model, so that there are always 2 OBGYN hospitalists on service. This strategy allows for the fellow to function as one of the hospitalists on-call, with the second hospitalist available to supervise, teach, and determine clinical competency in addition to other clinical responsibilities. Another option is to require the fellow to take call alongside another attending hospitalist for the first few months of fellowship, or until the fellow demonstrates clinical competency in various domains.

One final consideration is flexibility in clinical training, which allows programs to adapt the training experience to the clinical needs of the fellow. For example, some fellows may want more exposure to obstetric anesthesia if their desire is to practice abroad in remote locations. Others may desire more ultrasonography, critical care, or family planning experience. These are just a couple of ways in which a fellowship program can tailor training to the needs of their fellows.

THE BIGGEST CHALLENGE IN STARTING AND MAINTAINING AN OBGYN HOSPITALIST FELLOWSHIP

By and large, the biggest challenge in starting and maintaining a fellowship is recruitment. The ideal fellowship candidate will have career aspirations of becoming a leader in OBGYN hospital medicine and have a passion for education, patient safety, and simulation. Many programs have been successful at recruiting a senior resident from the same institution, but attracting applicants from elsewhere has proved more difficult. The primary reasons for this are national lack of awareness regarding the existence of OBGYN hospitalist fellowships and unfamiliarity with the benefits of fellowship training.

To combat this, fellowship directors will attempt to network and promote the fellowship at various academic conferences throughout the year. Others have taken the time to reach out to residency program directors directly, and some utilize social media to attract potential applicants. Nevertheless, the number of applicants applying each year remains low, which is additionally influenced by a difficult decision for residency graduates to defer attending-level salary for 1 to 2 years of fellowship training. As mentioned previously, the demand for OBGYN hospitalists is continuing to rise, and it is possible for graduates to be hired as a hospitalist right out of residency, especially for less competitive positions.

SUMMARY AND THE FUTURE OF OBGYN HOSPITALIST FELLOWSHIPS

In summary, OBGYN hospitalist fellowships were developed to train the future leaders of hospital medicine and inpatient clinician experts. To address the current supply and demand problem facing our specialty, these training programs can help recent residency graduates improve their confidence and competency in managing high-risk and emergent cases in OBGYN, as well as learn essential hospitalist skills not typically taught in residency, such as quality improvement, simulation, and leadership. In addition, fellows may have the opportunity to obtain advanced degrees as part of their training.

Similar to Minimally Invasive Gynecology and Pediatric and Adolescent Gynecology, which both evolved from the Generalist OBGYN Specialty and obtained a focused practice designation, OBGYN hospitalist fellowships may have the opportunity to do the same. One important step toward this will involve standardizing training across programs, an initiative that is currently the top priority of the SOGH Fellowship Committee. In the meantime, those desiring to start new fellowship programs are encouraged to utilize the SOGH Core Competencies and ACGME fellowship requirements as a basis for curriculum development. As fellowship programs continue to expand across the country, particular importance will need to be paid to recruitment and improving awareness regarding the importance of training the future leaders in OBGYN hospital medicine.

CLINICS CARE POINTS

- OBGYN hospitalists can improve the primary cesarean delivery rate (as well as nulliparous term singleton vertex cesarean delivery rate),[4–6] increase the likelihood of successful vaginal birth after cesarean, decrease rates of preterm births,[7] reduce the number of malpractice claims, lessen the incidence of critical safety events,[8,9] enhance resident and medical student education,[10] improve rates of severe maternal morbidity,[11] and close the gap in racial disparities in care.[12]

- Since the early 2000s, there has been a steady decline in the national average of many core OBGYN procedures performed by graduates from programs with accreditation from the Accreditation Council of Graduate Medical Education (ACGME).[3]

- Graduating residents are perceived to have deficits in professionalism, independent practice, psychomotor skills, clinical evaluation, and academic scholarship.

ACKNOWLEDGMENTS

The authors acknowledge the support provided by Phillip Bressman, MD—University of Tennessee, Ascension St. Thomas Hospital Midtown; Jennifer Butler, MD—University of California, Irvine; Brigid McCue, MD—Donald and Barbara Zucker School of Medicine at Hofstra/Northwell; and Kristin Powell, MD—University of Colorado.

DISCLOSURE

No financial conflicts of interest exist.

REFERENCES

1. Baudendistel T, Wachter R. The evolution of the hospitalist movement in the USA. Clin Med 2002;2(4):327–30.
2. McCue B, Shirillo A. OB/GYN hospitalist medicine: a review of the first decade of hospital focused practice. JOGHM Sept 2021;1(1):6–10.
3. Tatsis V, Butler J. Implementation of an academic OB/GYN hospitalist fellowship program: A sustainable training model for labor and delivery. J Gynecol Reprod Med 2018;2(1):1–4.
4. Iriye BK, Huang WH, Condon J, et al. Implementation of a laborist program and evaluation of the effect upon cesarean delivery. Am J Obstet Gynecol 2013; 209(3):251.e1-6.
5. Rosenstein MG, Nijagal M, Nakagawa S, et al. The association of expanded access to a collaborative midwifery and laborist model with cesarean delivery rates. Obstet Gynecol 2015;126(4):716–23.
6. Nijagal MA, Kuppermann M, Nakagawa S, et al. Two practice models in one labor and delivery unit: association with cesarean delivery rates. Am J Obstet Gynecol 2015;212(4):491.e1-8.
7. Srinivas SK, Small DS, Macheras M, et al. Evaluation the impact of the laborist model of obstetric care on maternal and neonatal outcomes. Am J Obstet Gynecol 2016;215(6):770.
8. Grunebaum A, Chervenak F, Skupski D. Effect of a comprehensive obstetric patient safety program on compensation payments and sentinel events. Am J Obstet Gynecol 2011;204:97–105.
9. Pettker CM, Thung SF, Lipkind HS, et al. A comprehensive obstetric patient safety program reduces liability claims and payments. Am J Obstet Gynecol 2014;211: 319–25.
10. Hauer KE, Wachter RM, McCulloch CE, et al. Effects of hospitalist attending physicians on trainee satisfaction with teaching and with internal medicine rotations. Arch Intern Med 2004;164:1866–71.
11. Torbenson V, Tatsis V, Bradley S, et al. Use of obstetric and gynecologic hospitalists is associated with decreased severe maternal morbidity in the United States. Patient Saf 2023;19:202–10.
12. Racial disparities in maternal outcomes: An analysis of the impact of OB hospitalist involved care on implicit bias. In: OBHG. 2023. Available at: https://obhg.com/wp-content/uploads/2023/04/OBHG-Race-data-analysis-1.pdf. [Accessed 1 October 2023].
13. Vintzileos A. Obstetrics and gynecology hospitalist fellowships. Obstet Gynecol Clin N Am 2015;42:541–8.
14. Funk C, Anderson BL, Schulkin J, et al. Survey of obstetric and gynecologic hospitalists and laborists. Am J Obstet Gynecol 2010;203. 177. e1-e4.
15. Gupta N, Dragovic K, Trester R, et al. The changing scenario of obstetrics and gynecology residency training. J Grad Med Educ 2015;401–6.
16. Guntupalli SR, Doo DW, Guy M, et al. Preparedness of obstetrics and gynecology residents for fellowship training. Obstet Gynecol 2018;126:559–68.

Obstetrician-Gynecologist Hospitalists as Educators

Sheila Hill, MD[a],*, Sara Carranco, MD[b,1],
Andrea LugoMorales, MD[b,2], William F. Rayburn, MD, MBA[c]

KEYWORDS

- Education • Competency/competencies • Hospitalist • Learning
- Obstetrician-gynecologist • Teaching

KEY POINTS

- The obstetrics and gynecology (ob/gyn) hospitalist position involves many opportunities for educating. Adaptive learning can take place in a range of contexts and situations.
- The ob/gyn hospitalist role in education is essential to the future growth of highly trained, exemplary ob/gyn hospitalists in both an academic and community hospital setting.
- Several learning formats can be utilized to educate about the roles and decision-making of hospitalists. Examples are cited.
- Development of educational competencies for ob/gyn hospitalists will aid in training of future hospitalists in community-based and academic settings.
- The ob/gyn hospitalist serves a pivotal role in the standardization of teaching and evidence-based practice in community-based and academic settings.

INTRODUCTION

The term hospitalist was first used to describe a new of type of United States physician by Wachter and Goldman in 1996.[1] Since the inception of the initial hospitalist movement in the early 1980s, the term hospitalist has grown with the current inclusionary group having academic and community spheres; primary care, specialty physicians, and advanced practice providers. The initial primary focus of the hospitalist was on the care of the hospitalized patient and quality and safety, but the authors have seen an expansion of this to include many roles and duties. Messler & Whitcomb

[a] Division of Hospitalist Medicine, Department of Obstetrics & Gynecology, Baylor College of Medicine, Texas Children's Pavilion for Women, 6651 Main Street, Suite 1060, Houston, TX 77030, USA; [b] Department of Obstetrics & Gynecology, Baylor College of Medicine, Houston, TX 77030, USA; [c] Department of Obstetrics and Gynecology, Medical University of South Carolina, 268 Calhoun Street, Charleston, SC 29425, USA
[1] Present address: 7600 Kirby Drive, Apartment 474, Houston, TX 77030.
[2] Present address: 4612 Chartres Street, Houston, TX 77004.
* Corresponding author. 64 Somerton Drive, Montgomery, TX 77356.
E-mail address: Sheila.hill@bcm.edu

Obstet Gynecol Clin N Am 51 (2024) 503–515
https://doi.org/10.1016/j.ogc.2024.06.001
0889-8545/24/© 2024 Elsevier Inc. All rights reserved, including those for text and data mining, AI training, and similar technologies.

give an excellent review of the progression of hospital medicine and its growth, initially mostly performed by internal medicine and pediatric colleagues to the solidification and the focus of the obstetrics and gynecology (ob/gyn) hospitalist.

In 2011 the Society of OB/GYN Hospitalists (SOGH)[2] was founded to support an ob/gyn hospitalist model, which promoted the values of excellence, collaboration, leadership, quality, and community in the care of women.[3] The SOGH defines an ob/gyn hospitalist as "the clinical experts for obstetric management and gynecologic emergencies" and the term *laborist as* "an ob/gyn who cares for obstetric patients on Labor and Delivery."[3] Since most ob/gyn hospitalists function beyond the Labor and Delivery unit, the term ob/gyn hospitalist is preferred. The American College of Obstetrics and Gynecology (ACOG) expands this definition to include the ob/gyn who has minimal outpatient and elective surgical responsibilities, and whose primary role is to care for hospitalized obstetric patients and to help manage obstetric emergencies that occur in the hospital. They may also provide urgent gynecologic care and consultation to the emergency department or hospital inpatient services.[4]

ROLES AND DUTIES OF THE OBSTETRICS AND GYNECOLOGY HOSPITALIST

Various employment models: employment with a hospital's physician network or contracted hospitalist group, self-contracted employment or member of an academic institution will define the framework of the various roles and duties of the ob/gyn hospitalist. The ob/gyn hospitalist often faces challenging, multi-faceted roles in a fast paced and dynamic environment. This may include clinical duties enhancing overall patient standard of care, administrative functions contributing to quality and safety initiatives, operational protocols, and information technology. The ob/gyn hospitalist provides availability and personalized care to patients and excels in critical event recognition. There is demonstrated research indicating improved maternal and neonatal outcomes such as reduced cesarean section rates and reduced maternal mortality.[5–7] The ob/gyn hospitalist plays a pivotal role in modern health care, contributing to the standardization of care across various medical specialties. Their presence ensures that patients receive consistent and evidence-based treatment promoting better outcomes. Regardless of the ob/gyn hospitalists' model of employment and whether they function in a large urban, academic, community or rural setting, a major focus of the ob/gyn hospitalist of the future will be on education (**Box 1**).

TRAINING OF THE OBSTETRICS AND GYNECOLOGY HOSPITALIST

In the past, internal medicine and pediatric training programs championed the development of both training programs to teach hospitalists how to improve health care quality and patient safety (PS), and how to attain established competencies.[8,9] In 2012 the Physician Leadership Forum of the American Hospital Association and the Society for Hospital Medicine hosted a half-day session at their Leadership Summit exploring how hospital-based medicine is evolving to re-shape care delivery in the hospital of the future. They focused on how the hospital-focused practice impacted delivery of care and practice could lead to better performance and safer hospital care.

Standardization in the tasks and roles of sub-specialty groups were looked at, referencing the SOGH as a dedicated society with resources available to facilitate these goals for the ob/gyn hospitalist.[10] Ob/gyn hospitalists are mainly comprised of board-certified practicing ob/gyn. This includes practitioners who have been in practice for many years to those just graduating from ob/gyn residency programs and who are seeking a specific lifestyle. Nationally, there are currently 11 ob/gyn hospitalist fellowship programs. SOGH is promoting ongoing discussion between the Accreditation

---

Box 1
The clinical roles and duties of the obstetrics and gynecology hospitalist

- Care of unassigned inpatient obstetric and gynecologic patients
- Provide triage or obstetric ED services
- Gynecologic consultation for hospitalized patients and the main emergency departments
- Oversight of residents, fellows, midwives, or advanced practice nurses
- Provide call coverage and labor and delivery support:
  - Interpretation of electronic fetal monitor strips
  - Stand-by for deliveries
  - Perform amniotomies and sonograms
  - IUPC/FSC placement
  - Monitoring of laboring patients for the private Obstetrician
- Maternal Fetal Medicine extenders
- Function as a member of and leader of the OB Rapid Response Team
- Surgically assist for other obstetricians or gynecologists
- Serve on patient safety and quality review committees
- Enforce quality metrics and evidence-based medicine

Abbreviations: ED, emergency department; IUPC, intrauterine fetal monitor/fetal monitor/fetal scalp electrode; OB, obstetrician; Ob/Gyn, obstetrician/gynecologist.

Council on Graduate Medical Education and ACOG with efforts to obtain ob/gyn hospital medicine as a focused practice designation. Part of this focus includes the development of standardized practices and competencies for ob/gyn hospitalists in practice, as well as those entering hospitalist fellowship programs.

SOGH has defined core competencies to encourage ob/gyn hospitalists to master a unique set of proficiencies. Core competencies are divided into 3 groups: Clinical Conditions, Health Systems, and Procedures. Each competency is then defined by its basic knowledge, skills, self-awareness/collaborative attitudes, system organization, and improvement.[3] Core competencies delineate the proficiencies required to function effectively as an ob/gyn hospitalist. They do not assess competence but rather establish standards expected of competent hospitalists in ob/gyn.

With the division of office-based practice and ob/gyn hospitalist practices, consideration must be given to maintenance of the ob/gyn privileges and competencies. The office-based practitioner may not be able to maintain competence in obstetric procedural skills and likewise the ob/gyn hospitalist competence in office practice skills and major gynecologic surgeries. The delineation of competencies will become crucial to standardized, safe, and evidence-based patient care.

THE OBSTETRICS AND GYNECOLOGY HOSPITALIST AS AN EDUCATOR

Much literature exists about the clinical, quality, operational, and administrative roles of the ob-gyn hospitalist. With the thrust of more hospitalist-based practice over the last several decades, the role of the hospitalist as an essential component of quality inpatient care has become tantamount. There has been a progression of hospitalist interactions with hospital administrative and ancillary staff, as well as development of quality health initiatives and protocol development, with their focus being on excellent, quality, and equitable patient care.

Whether a medical doctor acknowledges it or not, they are educators at some level. The expansion of the ob/gyn hospitalist originating in smaller community hospitals to larger academic centers has led to further development of their role as an educator. They not only care for the patient independently, decreasing the load on medicine teams, but have embraced the role of becoming effective educators.[11] While not at the forefront of ob/gyn hospitalist medicine, the value of the hospitalist as an essential educator in both community-based and academic centers is now more appreciated. Hospitalists play a vital role in education, providing valuable mentorship to peers, residents, and medical students. Their expertise contributes to the professional development of current and the next generation of health care providers, fostering a culture of continuous learning. The growth of programs in the community and academic settings has established the interprofessional and bi-directional nature of educational roles of the ob/gyn hospitalist between patients and family, community-based peers, nursing, ancillary, and administrative staff, as well as the academic program and clerkship director (**Fig. 1**). Larger urban and academic centers have the advantage of an in-house physician available for teaching to medical students, residents, and fellows. The performance of hospitalists has been studied in resident and medical student education in internal medicine and pediatric programs with an overall positive perception that the hospitalist is thought to be equal or better than the non-hospitalist in teaching value.[12] In addition, they are championed as fostering resident independence, supporting decision-making, teaching critical thinking, and providing feedback.[12] Whether a smaller community or large academic environment, the down-stream result of the ob/gyn hospitalist educator is highly trained, exemplary physicians who fulfill their various roles while providing quality, evidence-based, and equitable patient care.

The role of the ob/gyn hospitalist as educator should be held to definitive standards. In 2017 the SOGH Board of Directors established the Core Competencies Leadership Committee, which was to oversee and manage the preparation and planning for the development of core competencies for the ob/gyn hospitalist. The goal was to develop curricula for educating and training current and future hospitalists.

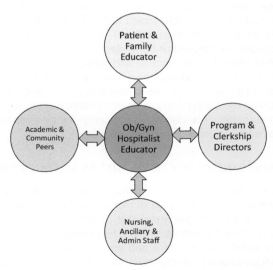

Fig. 1. Interprofessional multi-disciplinary educational roles of the ob/gyn hospitalists.

The final compilation was published in 2022 on a web-based educational platform. As a part of this compilation, a specific competency for the ob/gyn hospitalist as educator was developed.[13] **Table 1** is an adaption of this competency listing standards the ob/gyn hospitalist should demonstrate to be an effective educator. The SOGH has continued to regularly review and update these competencies, thus, providing an excellent resource for education and training of the ob/gyn hospitalist.

Teaching the Teacher

It is important to approach education in new and innovative ways and consider how hospitalists are "taught" to be teachers. An ob/gyn hospitalist who has been in practice for many years, serving in a community hospital can draw on a wealth of experience to share with peers. The younger ob/gyn hospitalist with definitive teaching competencies is an excellent resource for community hospital peers to help with educational programs within the hospital such as evidence-based updates. In an academic setting, an institution may provide training programs, which focus on the teacher or learner relationship. The Department of Education and Innovative Technology here at Baylor College of Medicine offers an 8-week Basic Educator Course to

Table 1 Educational competencies of the obstetrics and gynecology (Ob/Gyn) hospitalist as recommended by The Society of Ob/Gyn Hospitalists	
Knowledge	• Describe the role of Ob/Gyn Hospitalists as educators in different clinical environments • In academic settings, describe the ACGME educational goals for medical students, residents and fellows • Describe various models for teaching in the clinical setting • Discuss the benefits to trainees of pursing an Ob/Gyn hospital medicine fellowship • Discuss the role of simulation as an educational tool and explain the components of high-quality simulation
Skills	• Develop educational curricula and tools • Apply principles of adult learning to the educational process • Design education materials and session appropriate for learners experience level and knowledge • Plan the timing and delivery of information and learning experience • Communicate clear expectations and objectives • Use simulation as a teaching modality • Lead sessions on team-based learning • Serve as a role model and mentor for learners in the field of Ob/Gyn hospital medicine
Self-Awareness/ Collaborative Attitudes	• Embrace and value the role of educator, mentor and role model • Foster a work environment in which knowledge gaps are identified and addressed • Seek formal and informal feedback from learners and incorporate for improvement of teaching style and effectiveness
System Organizations & Improvement	• Advocate at the local, regional or national levels for programs and initiatives that support the continued professional develop of Ob/Gyn hospitalists as educators • Advance safety and quality improvement education in the field of Ob/Gyn hospital medicine

Adapted from The Society of Ob/Gyn Hospitalist Competencies.[13]

faculty. The course focuses on the inclusive learning environment within the framework of backward design, learner-centered assessment, and learner-centered teaching. The curriculum engages the teacher on how to make the learning environment equitable and accessible, how to design the curriculum to achieve meaningful outcomes, how assessments of learning align with outcome, how this information for feedback and evaluations is used, and how teaching can be active, addressing the needs of every student.

Teaching the Learner

With the increasing complexity, volume, technology, and amount of material to cover in medical education, it is essential to have many options in a hospitalist's armamentarium as educators. They must be aware of the many ways in which learners learn and be both direct and creative in teaching endeavors. While counterparts in internal medicine and pediatrics may have pioneered some of these educational methods in hospitalist medicine, the ob/gyn hospitalist has a unique challenge in that they must employ these educational methods in an often fast-paced, unpredictable environment.

Learning formats are numerous and must be individually applied. As educators, it is necessary to move away from the traditional didactic lecture and the "see one, do one, teach one" scenario. Thinking much more broadly about what the hospitalist is teaching and that it cannot be just "taught" but must be "caught" by the authors' learners. Additionally, the more non-traditional topics of patient advocacy, respectful care, PS, quality metrics, and professionalism require special attention.

Today's learners are different from those in the past, and networking and collaborative learning play important roles. With the use of modern technologies and e-learning, an almost infinite range of experiences can be provided for ob-gyn hospitalists to serve as teachers to address their peers' individual needs. Adaptive learning can take place in a range of contexts and situations–the classroom, triage areas, bedside, Labor and Delivery, operating room, or ward. The most effective learning depends on the context and mix or balance that varies at the different stages of training.

LEARNING FORMATS

The environment of the ob-gyn hospitalist offers many opportunities for teaching. The choice of learning format or teaching method depends on several perspectives: expected learning outcomes, tools to be used, context or location where the learning is situated, educational strategies to be adopted, and special needs of the learners. Briefly described as follows are different learning formats to be used for professional development. More detailed descriptions about each format may be read elsewhere.[14] **Table 2** highlights examples used by the ob-gyn hospitalist.

On-the-Job or Work-Based Experience

Learning from experience is fundamental in acquiring the knowledge, skills, and dispositions required for practice and in maintaining competence. Learning on the job is responsible for perhaps as much as 70% of professional learning with formal workshops and training accounting for only 10%.[15] Likewise, faculties mostly learn about teaching directly from teaching experiences and from colleagues rather than faculty developers.[16] A key understanding principle is that learning is inherent in everyday practice through taking responsibility, being actively involved, and interacting with colleagues of the team. There are many examples of this type of learning, which include labor board huddles, rounding on patients, and one-to-one procedure performance.

Table 2
Examples of specific learning formats used by Ob/GYn hospitalists

Learning Format	Examples
On-the-job experience	Hands on ultrasound training
	Patient rounds
	Patient sign-out
Small group sessions	Debrief sessions
	Group patient rounding
	Patient care huddles
Lecturers/conferences	SOGH Annual Clinical Meeting
	Grand rounds
	Morbidity and Mortality Conferences
	Multi-disciplinary conferences
Simulations	Post-partum hemorrhage
	Hypertensive emergency
	Massive transfusion protocol
Online resources	Up-to-Date
	Google Scholar
	Cochrane Data Base
	CDC STI Treatment
	Online textbooks and podcasts
Reflection	Debrief sessions
	Case reviews/clinical care conundrums
	Situational ethics
Peer observation/feedback	Clinical presentation feedback
	Surgical performance feedback
	Patient counseling feedback
Self-directed learning	Entrusting with mentor guidance
	Unguided self-reflection/reading
	Self-directed assessment
QI/PS projects	Data assessment cesarean section rates
	Post-procedural debriefs
	Resident projects
Checklists/protocols	Twin vaginal delivery checklist
	Hypertensive emergency checklist
	Suicide screening
	Placenta accreta spectrum screening
Communication skills	Peer-to-Peer communication
	Physician-to patient communication and feedback
	Resident patient interaction feedback
Professionalism	Peer-Peer interactions
	Peer feedback

Abbreviations: PS, patient safety; QI, quality improvement; SOGH, society of Ob/Gyn hospitalists.

Small Group Sessions

The value of small group teaching is well-recognized for problem-based learning. Each clinical encounter provides clues and suggestions that enable the clinician to learn what she or he needs to know and do. The setting can influence learning in inpatient wards, emergency department, operating rooms, Labor and Delivery, or anywhere a clinical encounter occurs between a clinician and patient. The context of a small group session includes people, processes, technology, and sociocultural influences. This type of learning can also lend itself to the ob/gyn hospitalist to peer education of evidence-based topics in a busy clinical setting. Web-based storage may also provide easy access to peers for future reference.

Lectures or Conferences

A formal, planned activity presents the stereotypical picture of a didactic lecture or conference and an array of professional participants engaged in the learning experience. These activities include a variety of formats: conferences (live or online), regularly scheduled series (ie, grand rounds), workshops, symposia, refresher courses, and enduring materials (printed or online). While lectures may not work to affect practice change or health care outcomes, they do offer a relatively efficient way of delivering educational content.[17] Lectures are less often attended in formal large settings and accessed more online at times available for the learner to be less distracted. Lectures have also been combined with hands on teaching such as an ultrasound conference with hands-on-scanning of patients.

Simulation

The potential in hospital care is tremendous for simulation-based education and training to enhance patient outcomes and promote PS. A variety of stimulations and simulators could be used effectively in innovative education and training models to address the spectrum of clinical skills, technical skills, nontechnical skills, and teamwork. Centers with learning opportunities using simulators and simulated patients are a feature of many institutions. Access to such facilities is now recognized through all phases of medical education. A variety of simulations are in existence and often used for training and teaching on an annual basis within the hospital environment. Despite the anticipated benefits, several challenges that need to be considered are cost, fidelity, and physician acceptance.

Online Resources and Computer Suites

The learning of most physicians and health care professionals is directed by patient encounters in the clinical environment. The sheer volume of medical literature bears witness to internet (or online) searches as playing a key role in answering clinical questions. The movement prompting additional information seeking is from having better informed patients, more patient comfort in searching this information, more pre-reviewed literature with changes in diagnosis and management, and information being more accessible at the provider's fingertips. Hospitals offer computer suites, and often multi-media resource areas, for individual or collaborative learning.

Reflection

Reflection by a clinician is well-recognized as a critical component of learning. Improving care requires not only a fund of practical knowledge accrued from formal education but also accumulated from past, similar experiences. Reflection usually involves some weighing of options, which usually leads to a decision on how to act at that time. The revisiting of evidence and extracting what has been learned can add to the physician's knowledge and confidence when applied again. In addition, most clinicians at some stage in their career will have prepared many lectures, run small group discussions, or counseled, which include reflecting on their performance in relation to the task.[17]

Peer Observation or Feedback

The combination of peer observation and feedback of patient management is becoming a more acceptable practice at many medical schools and hospital settings.

External feedback is a fundamental element in enhancing the accuracy of self-assessment. It is important that the feedback be constructive rather than destructive and preferably team-based. Feedback comes not only from peers but also from other sources: students, nurses, social workers, patients, and audits. Focusing on content and coaching for change holds promise of opportunities for physicians to respond to their feedback with a trusted peer or supervisor.[18]

Self-Directed Learning

In student-directed learning, the ob-gyn hospitalist has important roles in clarifying learning outcomes, assessing the learner's knowledge and skills, planning the most appropriate sequence and pace of learning, and advising about available learning resources to meet their personal needs.[19] Opportunity to engage with a coach would help learners create and stick to a plan, interpret the performance data to determine learning needs, identify evidence-based resources and select opportunities for learning, try out what was learned, and incorporate what was learned into routine practice.[20]

The development of a research thesis, design of a protocol, and execution of the project constitute a model of mentor engagement for self-directed learning.

Morbidity and Mortality Conferences

Morbidity and mortality is a major exemplar of an educational forum that seeks to integrate many aspects of health care quality and value. Highlighted are often systems issues, promoting evidence-based practice, and identifying quality improvement (QI) opportunities. Evidence to promote communication represents a rich opportunity for care improvement. Using a case-based, problem-based, and team-learning approach, this learning format encourages a more meticulous understanding and discussion about individual care. This experiential way of learning and promoting systems thinking leverages unique contributions using a multigenerational and multidisciplinary approach. Hospital committee such as Quality Assessment Performance Improvement Committees is an illustration that exemplifies this learning technique. Various patient cases are reviewed looking at deviation or variance from policy, procedures, or guidelines.

Quality Improvement or Patient Safety Projects

Failures in health care still occur. Improving quality of care and reducing adverse events are galvanizing forces for change. The ability to operationalize improvement efforts is in many ways more essential for physicians looking to successfully be part of, or run, patient care. Fundamentally, QI approaches consist of systematic and continuous actions that lead to measurable improvement in health care delivery to targeted patient groups. Commonly taught QI or PS skills include defining aims, measurements, identifying waste, process mapping, and conducting root cause analyses.

Checklist and Protocol Utilization

Active practitioners are inclined to keep checklists and follow protocols. A primary function of a checklist is documentation of the task for auditing or training when dealing with time-critical situations. Written checklists should focus on the responsibilities of a specific clinician or a group who will work together to avoid leaving out items and be more efficient and keep on track. Use of a well-designed checklist can reduce any tendency to avoid, omit, or neglect important steps in any task. Written protocols demonstrate an awareness of and responsiveness to the health care system and the ability to effectively call on system resources to provide care that is more consistent for optimal patient outcomes and safety. A checklist for post-partum discharge or women with hypertensive disorders used at the authors' institution is shown in **Fig. 2**.

Communication Skills

Effective communication between providers and with patients is an essential core competency to learn. The quality of interactions that patients experience in their care highly influences the positive or negative perception of the care they receive. Communication failures can be complex and relate to vertical hierarchical differences, concerns with upward influence, conflicting roles, and ambiguities, and struggles with interpersonal power. Learning by overcoming these barriers to effective communication, therefore, needs to be addressed constructively at the appropriate level. At the authors' institution, new faculties and physicians are offered a seminar "Breakthrough in Communication." The focus of the seminar is basic communication with patients, families, and colleagues and staff.

Checklist for Postpartum Discharge of Women with Hypertensive Disorders

1/10/2022

Follow-up

☐ Ensure patient has contact information for obstetrical provider (phone, electronic patient portal).
☐ Ensure patient has scheduled follow-up (in-person or telehealth).
    o Patients with the following should have a schedule office visit/telehealth[a] for BP check within 3-5 days of discharge (ideally within 72 hours):
        ▪ Received rapid-acting antihypertensive medication(s) during delivery hospitalization
        ▪ Preeclampsia with severe features (including superimposed)
        ▪ Eclampsia
    o All other patients should have a scheduled office visit/telehealth[a] for BP check at 7 to 10 days after delivery

☐ Evaluate and address barriers to care, such as:
    o   Transportation and childcare for visit(s)
    o   Access to telephone if needed to call provider or reschedule appointments
    o   Access to interpretation services if needed
    o   Resources to fill/pick up prescription(s)
    o   **If any barriers are identified, consult Social Work prior to discharge**

☐ If patient has home blood pressure cuff:
    o   Provide instruction on how to measure blood pressure.
    o   Ensure literacy, ability to read and interpret numbers
    o   Review frequency of home BP monitoring: patients should take BP 1-2 times daily after discharge until at least 7-10 days postpartum.
    o   Discuss target blood pressures (systolic less than 150 mm Hg; diastolic less than 100 mm Hg).
    o   Discuss blood pressures requiring prompt notification (systolic 160 mm Hg or greater; diastolic 110 mm Hg or greater).

☐ Create a postpartum check-in plan for the first 2-3 weeks postpartum:
    o   Ask mother to identify 1 or 2 people who can call her at least once daily after discharge from the hospital if she will be home alone.
    o   Advise mother and family to post emergency contact information in a readily available place at home; make sure key family members are aware.

Fig. 2. Texas Children's Hospital checklist for postpartum discharge of women with hypertensive disorders. [a]Telehealth visits are only appropriate if the patient has a home blood pressure cuff upon discharge. (*Adapted from* SMFM Special Statement: Checklist for Postpartum discharge for women with hypertensive disorders.)

Professionalism

More physicians are now employed by hospitals or health care systems. The hospitalist is a role model of professionalism. Professionalism can be taught directly or indirectly as a commitment to carrying out responsibilities, adhering to ethical principles, and being sensitive to a diverse patient population and social determinants of health. An important aspect of the transition to professionalism has been the daily shift toward population health and the inclusion of public health concepts. Health care professionals will be required to be engaged in integral parts of the whole system and continuous quality improvement to attain better outcomes, efficiencies, and cost-containment.

SUMMARY AND FUTURE DIRECTION

The progressive growth of the hospitalist model of practice over the past 20 years has solidified the role of the ob/gyn hospitalists as an essential component of quality inpatient care. The ob/gyn hospitalist as an educator is proving to be a tantamount role in the future. The ob/gyn hospitalist's role as an educator has long-term benefits and implications for the standardization of education and evidence-based patient care both in the community-based and academic practice settings.

Growth of artificial intelligence (AI) in various fields, especially medicine and education, has many implications for hospitalists and other health professionals. As AI tools become increasingly used in health care delivery, ob-gyn hospitalists will need to be competent in their optimal use and limitations. As educators, hospitalists will need to understand how generative AI tools, such as ChatGPT and Bard, have the potential to revolutionize any hospital where creation and innovation are the keys. Applications, including self-directed learning, simulation scenarios, and writing assistance must be carefully balanced with issues of academic integrity, data accuracy, and potential detriments for learning.[21]

The future training of the ob/gyn hospitalists will likely include the demonstration of competencies in not only clinical practice skills but also in basic knowledge, self-awareness or collaborative attitudes, system organization, and improvement. Through educational opportunities, ob/gyn hospitalists will grow as vital resources for advancing PS and high-quality care.

CLINICS CARE POINTS

- The steady expansion in community hospitals, increased presence within academic centers, and development of fellowship programs have led to increased opportunities for ob/gyn hospitalists to serve as educators.
- The clinical duties of ob/gyn hospitalists vary depending on clinical setting, yet they are a valuable educational resource in any program.
- Examples of learning formats include teaching teamwork and communication skills through simulation, partnering with clinical nurse educators to implement new protocols, facilitating formal didactics, or teaching hands-on skills to students, residents, new staff, and peers.
- A significant role of the ob/gyn hospitalist is as an educator in the patient-physician relationship, ensuring that patients are informed and engaged in their care.
- As educational leaders, ob/gyn hospitalists serve as vital resources for advancing PS and high-quality care.

ACKNOWLEDGMENTS

Course Developers, Department of Education and Innovative Technology, Baylor College of Medicine for review of their Basic Educators Course.

DISCLOSURE

Express our gratitude to Dr. Charles Kilpatrick, Baylor College of Medicine for critical review of this article.

REFERENCES

1. Wachter RM, Goldman L. The emerging role of "hospitalists" in the American health care system. N Engl J Med 1996;335:514–7.
2. Messler J, Whitcomb WF. A history of the hospitalist movement. Obstet Gynecol Clin N Am 2015;46:419–32.
3. SOGH Website. Available at: https://societyofobgynhospitalist.org/faqs-for-prospective-ob-byn-hospitalist/. [Accessed 9 January 2024].
4. ACOG Committee Opinion. The obstetric and gynecologic hospitalist. Obstet Gynecol 2016;127(2):e81–5.
5. Iriye B. Impact of obstetrician/gynecologist hospitalists on quality of obstetric care (Cesarean delivery rates, trial of labor after Cesarean/vaginal birth after Cesarean rates, and neonatal adverse events). Obstet Gynecol Clin N Am 2015;42: 477–85.
6. Stevens T, Swaim L, Clark S. The role obstetrics/gynecology hospitalists in reducing maternal mortality. Obstet Gynecol Clin N Am 2015;42:463–75.
7. Torbenson V, Tatsis V, Bradley S, et al. Use of obstetric and gynecologic hospitalists is associated with decreased severe maternal morbidity in the United States. J Patient Saf 2023;19(3):202–10.
8. O'Leary KJ, Afsar-Manesh N, Budnitz T, et al. Hospital quality and patient safety competencies: development, description, and recommendations for use. J Hosp Med 2011;6:530–6.
9. Lubrizzi J, Winer J, Banach L, et al. Perceived core competency achievements of fellowship and non-fellowship-trained early career hospitalists. J Hosp Med 2015; 6:373–9.
10. Proceedings from American Hospital Association Health Forum/Leadership Summit July. Creating the hospital of the future: implications of hospital-focused physician practice | AHA 2012. [Accessed 19 January 2024].
11. Liston B, O'Dorisio N, Walker C, et al. Hospital medicine in the internal medicine clerkship: results from a national survey. J Hosp Med 2012;7(7):557–61.
12. Heydarian C, Maniscalco J. Pediatric hospitalists in medical education: current roles and future directions. Curr Probl Pediatr Adolesc Health Care 2012;42: 120–6.
13. SOGH Ob/Gyn Resource Center, Ob/gyn hospitalists' core competencies. Available at: Table of Contents | SOGH Resource Center (unboundmedicine.com). [Accessed January 25, 2024].
14. Rayburn WF, Turco MG, Davis DA, editors. Continuing professional development in medicine and health care. Better education, better patient outcomes. Philadelphia, PA: Wolters Kluwer; 2018.
15. Jennings C, Wargnier J. Effective Learning with 70:20:10; Cross Knowledge. 2011. Available at: http://www.crossknowledge/whitepapers/effective-learning-with-70_20_10-whitepaper.pdf. [Accessed 25 December 2023].

16. Oleson A, Hora MT. Teaching the way they were taught? Revisiting the sources of teaching knowledge and the role of prior experience in shaping faculty teaching practices. High Educ 2013;68:29–45.

17. Forsetlund I, Bjorndal A, Rashidian A, et al. Continuing education meetings and workshops: effects on professional practice and health care outcomes. Cochrane Database Syst Rev 2009;2:CD003030.

18. Sargeant J, Lockyer J, Mann K, et al. Facilitated reflective performance feedback: developing an evidence and theory-based model that builds relationships, explores reactions and content, and coaches for performance change (R2C2). Acad Med 2015;90:1698–706.

19. Sargeant J. Toward a mutual understanding of self-assessment. J Contin Educ Health Prof 2008;28:1–4.

20. Lyasere C, Baggett M, Romano J, et al. Beyond continuing medical education: clinical coaching as a tool for ongoing professional development. Acad Med 2016;91:1647–50.

21. Preiksaitis C, Rose C. Opportunities, challenges, and future directions of generative artificial intelligence in medical education: scoping review. JMIR Med Educ 2023;9:e48785.

Obstetrics and Gynecology Hospitalists as Champions of Drills and Simulation

Lisbeth M. McKinnon, MD[a,b,1], Eileen M. Reardon, MD[c,*]

KEYWORDS

- Simulation-based education • Obstetric and gynecologic simulation
- Ob/gyn hospitalist • Quality improvement

KEY POINTS

- Obstetrics and gynecology (Ob/Gyn) Hospitalists play an essential role in advocating for and leading obstetric and gynecologic simulation-based education and emergency drills.
- Ob/Gyn Hospitalists are champions for quality and safety using a variety of types of simulation modalities.
- Simulation training, education, and leadership are valuable skills of a proficient Ob/Gyn Hospitalist.

INTRODUCTION

The rapidly growing field of obstetrics and gynecologist (Ob/Gyn) Hospitalist Medicine has contributed to the improved quality of care of birthing persons.[1,2] As well as being the first responders to emergency situations, Ob/Gyn Hospitalists play a key role in maintaining the overall quality and safety of care in their institutions.[3] Because of this unique focus, it was logical that Ob/Gyn Hospitalists would welcome and integrate simulation-based education as a useful tool to optimize patient safety and outcomes. Although the specific duties of the Ob/Gyn Hospitalist may vary from hospital to hospital, one role that never varies is the call to the emergent patient situation. It is fortunate that the most serious situations are infrequent but when they do happen, a practiced and efficient team response will help ensure the best outcome. Through simulation activities, the Ob/Gyn Hospitalist can learn and maintain clinical skills, hone teamwork skills such as communication and situational awareness, and play an active role in the overall safety and quality of care in their hospitals.[4,5]

[a] Overlake Medical Center, Bellevue, WA, USA; [b] Ob-Hospitalist Group, Greenville, SC, USA; [c] Intermountain Health, Peaks Region, Denver, CO, USA
[1] Present address: 13009 230th Avenue Southeast, Issaquah, WA 98027.
* Corresponding author.
E-mail address: Ereardonmd.co@gmail.com

Obstet Gynecol Clin N Am 51 (2024) 517–525
https://doi.org/10.1016/j.ogc.2024.05.006 **obgyn.theclinics.com**

Definitions and Terms

The terms "Simulation" and "Drill" are sometimes used interchangeably and the difference may be a matter of semantics. A drill is a practice exercise for a rare but critical event; it is often used by institutions when testing a process. The term "simulation" has a more educational overtone with a more formal structure and is used in courses and seminars.[6] Although simulation can be applied to any educational area, our discussion and use of Simulation-based Education, or simply Simulation, will be restricted to simulation in the health care setting.

Skill-based simulation (eg, forceps training) and immersive simulation (practicing a complex situation — eg, management of a rare emergency condition) have been used for over 250 years. This was not only a way to reduce the chance of harm to a patient but was also used in areas where there was limited patient population.[6] After a marked decline in the twentieth century, simulation as an educational staple has recently enjoyed a resurgence in medical schools, health care systems, and national conferences. A major impetus was The Institute of Medicine's groundbreaking publication: To Err Is Human: Building a Safer Health System (1999).[7] This study revealed that up to 80% of obstetric sentinel events could be traced to deficiencies in the process of team skills, with the most common being inadequate communication. Simulation is one of the most effective tools utilized to address this deficiency. Through simulation-based education, health care providers practice and maintain nonclinical skills such as communication, situational awareness, and other teamwork concepts.

There are many ways to run simulation activities, and the method chosen should take into account readily available resources and facilities. It is not necessary to spend thousands on high-tech equipment to produce a quality simulation. An excellent cost-effective simulation can be produced by utilizing volunteer actors, low-tech home-made props and expired supplies. An example of a low-tech prop is a "uterus" made out of a ski hat, zipper, and furniture foam which can be used to teach or practice compression sutures for control of postpartum hemorrhage. See **Fig. 1**.

When developing a simulation or drill, fidelity is an important concept that heavily influences the educational experience.[8] Fidelity can refer to the degree of technical complexity; referring to the modality employed, the equipment and props used, or both. A tabletop simulation exercise is a low-fidelity group exercise that is a useful form of simulation. No props or actors are needed. The participants, often sitting around a table, run through a scenario as if it were happening in front of them. This

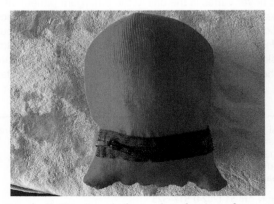

Fig. 1. Low-tech prop of a "uterus" made from a hat, furniture foam, and zipper for practicing compression sutures. (*Courtesy* Dr. Eileen M. Reardon.)

can be an effective tool to help with knowledge deficits, work out system issues, and standardize protocols.[9] A skill- based simulation is meant to teach or evaluate a particular skill, such as a pelvic trainer for practicing shoulder dystocia maneuvers. An immersive simulation is a simulated emergency exercise requiring participants to play the roles that would be encountered in a real life emergency. A typical simulation has a goal with defined objectives, a written scenario or script, a briefing, running the scenario, and a debriefing.[9,10] The patient and 1 or 2 roles are often played by volunteers. Including these embedded actors can help guide the other participants toward the learning goal, or provide distractions or confounders. These simulations often incorporate high-fidelity mannequins that have many "lifelike" functions: eye movement, voice capabilities, intravenous (IV) sites, the ability to bleed, have a cardiac arrest, etc. See **Fig. 2**.

Simulation using virtual technology can be used to reach a wider group of participants. There are high-tech virtual reality simulations throughout health care education, but a virtual simulation can also be created and run in a cost-effective manner. Using a smartphone camera, a group of volunteers can act out a simulation several times, with varying outcomes. The film can be clipped into small scenes or filmed that way initially. This can then be used on a web-based media platform with a multiple-choice question format. The participants' answers then trigger the next scene shown, and so on until the endpoint is reached.

"Fidelity," somewhat confusingly, is also the term used to describe another important simulation component: the perceived reality of the simulation scenario, props, and

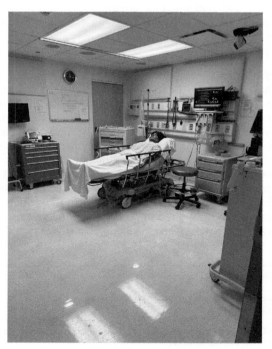

Fig. 2. Example of a simulation set-up in a simulation center room with a high-tech mannequin. (Reardon, E. 2021 Northwestern Simulation Center: Feinberg School of Medicine, Chicago, IL.)

environment.[6,8] Realism is an individual perception, and simulation educators must partner with their learners in what is often termed a *"fiction contract."*[11] A fiction contract is a collaborative agreement between educators and learners to treat the simulated environment as "real" while acknowledging the limitations. There are 3 defined concepts of fidelity. Physical fidelity is exactly that: the degree to which the learner's physical senses (sight, hearing, touch, etc) interpret the scenario as authentic. Conceptional fidelity is how plausible the scenario appears to the learner, that is, does this mimic/proceed along as a real life similar situation would? Emotional fidelity, also termed "experimental fidelity," is the degree to which the learner experiences the feelings they would have in a similar real patient case. These 3 kinds of fidelity influence the learner's perception of reality. A greater sense of reality and "buy-in" directly correlate with the success of achieving the education goals of the simulation[6,8] See **Fig. 3**.

Validation and Recognition of Simulation as a Tool for Developing and Maintaining Clinical Excellence and Patient Safety

Throughout the field of obstetrics and gynecology, there is widespread support and affirmation of the value of Simulation-based education. Several national leading organizations have stated their support for simulation-based education and training.

American College of Obstetrics and Gynecology
The American College of Obstetrics and Gynecology (ACOG) emphasizes the importance of simulation. In Committee Opinion 590 *Preparing for Clinical Emergencies in Obstetrics and Gynecology,* simulations and drills are recognized as key tools for optimal management and mitigation of emergency situations, along with Rapid Response Teams (RRT) and Early Warning Systems. Not only can the practice gained through simulation improve a team response, but it may also expose areas or aspects of care that need improvement.[2]

American Board of Obstetrics and Gynecology
The American Board of Obstetrics and Gynecology (ABOG) has its Maintenance of Certification Program in which all Board-Certified Obstetrician/Gynecologists must participate to maintain their status. One of required categories is termed "Practice Improvement Activities," commonly known as Part IV. Under the category of Quality Improvement/Simulation, participation in one of several national Emergency Simulation courses is an option for completing this requirement.[12]

Society of Obstetrics and Gynecology Hospitalists The Society of Ob/Gyn Hospitalists (SOGH) has developed the Core Competencies which "establish the standards expected of competent Ob/Gyn Hospitalists."[13] The Core Competencies for Ob and Ob/Gyn Hospitalists[13] were developed to "standardize the practice model, set goals for fellowship training, and better define the leadership role of hospitalists in women's

---

Physical fidelity: degree to which the simulation is sensed as "real".

Conceptual fidelity: degree to which the simulation proceeds in a causally plausible manner

Emotional fidelity: degree to which the simulation generates feelings that would arise in a real situation.

Fig. 3. Definitions of the types of fidelity in simulation-based exercises. (Reardon, E. Unpublished lecture Denver CO 2022.)

health." One of the Core Competencies is Simulation: it states: "As providers on the front lines, Ob/Gyn Hospitalists should be champions for simulation as a tool for achieving and maintaining safety and high-quality care in the hospital setting."[13] The document goes on to detail that the Ob/Gyn Hospitalist should be actively involved in promoting and running simulations. See **Fig. 4**.

The Joint Commission (TJC): In the United States, the top 2 causes of maternal morbidity and mortality are hypertensive disorders of pregnancy and hemorrhage. TJC, embracing the findings in *To Err is Human,* that is, that medical errors often result from communication breakdown between teams, modified their Perinatal Standards in 2019.[14] With the goal of increasing maternal safety, they added several Elements of Performance to their Perinatal Standards. Included was a requirement for all hospitals with labor and delivery departments to conduct regular (defined as at least annually) drills in these areas. Ob/Gyn Hospitalists across the country welcomed this as an opportunity to further impel the intregration of simulation into their hospitals.[14]

ROLES OF THE OB-GYN HOSPITALIST

The concept of Ob/Gyn Hospitalist championing simulation-based education and drills could well have been foreseen considering the breadth of skills, knowledge, responsibilities, and Core Competencies. The specific scope of clinical responsibilities of an Ob/Gyn Hospitalist varies amongst institutions. It is often defined by the needs of the particular hospital and of its community. The unique role of Ob/Gyn Hospitalists places them in a strategic position to help drills and simulations become an integral part of their hospital's policies, quality improvement processes, and team culture.

Ob/Gyn hospitalist medicine continues to expand and is rapidly evolving to have an ever increasing focus on safety. Ob/Gyn Hospitalists require the skill of situational awareness which aids in their overall support of the labor and delivery unit. They are in effect safety officers of the unit. They support community providers, midwives, family practitioners, maternal fetal medicine specialists, and nursing staff. They are physically present in the hospital at all times, ensuring availability of immediate emergency response which lends itself to strong and trusting relationships with staff. Simulation-based education activities provide an opportunity to engage all members of the

---

SOGH Core Competency: Simulation

OB/GYN hospitalists should be able to:

- Collaborate to design and run multidisciplinary simulation drills and encourage and facilitate participation by all members of the health care team.
- Seek out lifelong learning opportunities to maintain low-frequency, high-acuity skills.

OB/GYN hospitalists should be able to:

- Advocate for simulation as an integral part of quality assurance and process improvement initiatives, staff and resident education, patient safety initiatives, team training, and building a culture of safety.
- Identify opportunities for simulation and participate in simulation drills.
- Advocate for and support efforts to establish a standard of debriefing after near misses and adverse events.

Fig. 4. The society of obstetrics and gynecology (Ob/Gyn) hospitalists core competencies for the Ob and Ob/Gyn Hospitalist.[13]

patient care team in the practice of team building.[15] Important team building skills that can be targeted include communication, coordination of care, preparation, skill-building, and efficient emergency response.

Ob/Gyn Hospitalists often function as part of an institution's Obstetric rapid response team (RRT), sometimes referred to as the "OB Stat Team."[16] An RRT is a medical emergency team of multidisciplinary health care professionals with expertise in critical care who are trained to respond to emergencies. The key concept of an RRT is a team-oriented approach to prevent harm as soon as there are early signs of patient deterioration. RRTs have been utilized in the hospital setting since the 2000s. Obstetric- specific RRTs, termed "OB RRTs," are becoming more and more common. ACOG, TJC, Agency for healthcare Research and Quality, and the Association of Women's Health, Obstetric, and Neonatal Nurses all endorse development of RRT as a patient safety initiative. Ob/Gyn Hospitalists are repetitively involved in emergency responses and are considered experts in emergency. Almost all Ob/Gyn Hospitalists have experience in participation in simulations: through hospitalist organization, annual conferences (such as the Society of Ob/Gyn Hospitalists Annual Clinical Meeting Simulation Course), prior simulation experience during training, or other continuing educational simulation training. They are thus uniquely qualified to help develop, coordinate, and lead OB RRTs. Simulations provide an opportunity to practice team-approached emergency care drills which are critical in a competent OB RRT Team.[15,17]

The Ob/Gyn Hospitalist thus plays a critical role in helping provide optimal care across several disciplines. Communication and relationship building are key aspects of the role of a consultant. The Ob/Gyn Hospitalist often provides obstetric and gynecologic consultations for patients in the Emergency Department and on other inpatient services. In this respect, they partner with health care providers of several specialties. Especially in the critical or emergency situations, ensuring efficient teamwork among providers who do not regularly work together is a key component to optimal outcomes. Conducting interprofessional simulations provides a platform to practice this important skill.[18] Evolving from in-person gathering restrictions during the COVID pandemic, virtual simulations have provided an effective opportunity for large groups of health care workers to participate in interprofessional simulations remotely.

Ob/Gyn Hospitalists often support the Maternal Fetal Medicine (MFM) service. In many institutions, the Ob/Gyn Hospitalist service will partner with the MFM consultants, helping to admit and manage high-risk patients in the hospital. Working with MFMs, Ob/Gyn Hospitalists can develop and facilitate plans for high-risk patients, both for long-term care and acute obstetric emergency. A table top simulation is ideally suited for this, enabling members of the patient care team to walk through emergency scenarios step by step and discuss the steps they would take in a real-life event.

A common responsibility of the Ob/Gyn Hospitalist is providing obstetric emergency department (OBED) and triage coverage. In this setting, the Ob/Gyn Hospitalist may need to respond emergently to various critical obstetric situations. The success of an emergency response relies on strong leadership as well as prompt, efficient, and collaborative team skills. The opportunity to practice emergency obstetric situations with staff is a valuable tool in improving patient care and outcomes with the added benefit of improving team performance and confidence.[16] Some examples of emergency drills relevant to the OBED setting include placental abruption, uterine rupture in the evaluation of a patient presenting with abdominal pain, and severe hypertensive crisis where timely treatment is critical in lowering the risk of severe maternal morbidity.[19]

The presence of an Ob/Gyn Hospitalist assures unbiased quality care for all individuals that present to the hospital, including unassigned patients. An unassigned patient is any individual who presents to the hospital for care and treatment who has not established care with a provider. Some of these patients may be uninsured and have socioeconomic barriers to care. Diversity, equity, inclusion, and cultural competency are important nonclinical skills. These have been also called "soft skills" that is, personal qualities that facilitate communication and understanding. Hard skills refer to the more technical clinical skills. Both hard and soft skills are important in optimizing patient care. They can improve communication, increase empathy, and increase patient satisfaction. Soft skills can be learned by incorporating them into emergency simulation scenarios. This strategy has been effective in training hospital care teams in providing optimal care for a patient population they encounter infrequently.[6]

An important role of the Ob/Gyn Hospitalist is training and education. Many are involved in teaching and overseeing residents, medical students, and sometimes nursing students. Ob/Gyn Hospitalists play an important role in encouraging students and trainees to participate in simulations. Simulation-based education is an opportunity to learn in a safe non-judgmental environment where patients are not put at risk and their clinical skills can develop. Ob/Gyn Hospitalists can be drivers of change, championing team-building emergency drills encompassing of all members of the care team: residents, students, community providers, and nursing staff. In doing so, they can identify opportunities for learning and encourage creative approaches to simulation education.[9,20]

Ob/Gyn Hospitalists are leaders and advocates of patient safety initiatives. They are uniquely positioned to support quality metrics and support evidence-based medicine. They can help with establishing hospital quality initiatives, then achieving and enforcing these quality standards. Simulations can play an important role in achieving these goals. As already mentioned, simulations and drills are part of TJCrequirements for patient risk reduction strategies and are required as part of the elements of performance standards. In championing and leading simulation activities, Ob/Gyn Hospitalists can play an important role in advocating simulations in an effort to maintain hospital quality and compliance standards.[14]

Even with the widespread recognition of the value of simulation-based education and drills, championing and establishing them can have its challenges. Conducting regular simulations has become a common quality and safety expectation of hospitals across the nation yet there are still barriers to implementation. Time can be a factor, whether trying to work a drill into a busy shift or giving up personal time on an off day. Although nursing staff is routinely compensated for educational participation, that concept has rarely been applied to providers. Hospital systems are increasingly making these simulation activities mandatory for privileging but not offering compensation. The result is that physicians often end up taking clinic or surgery time to participate in a "voluntary" fashion. Similarly, Ob/Gyn Hospitalists are not often compensated for the even larger time commitment of developing and running these exercises. Medical staff colleagues may be reluctant to participate, not only because of time constraints and financial reasons detailed earlier but also from unfamiliarity with the value of these exercises. Limited organizational resources, additional financial constraints, and lack of administrative support may contribute to the difficulty.

Quality metrics, value-add services, and team coordination are all becoming more of a focus of health care systems. The simulation industry is rapidly growing alongside a rapidly growing field of Ob/Gyn hospitalist medicine. In the future, there will be even more established simulation training programs in hospital settings as quality outcomes continue to show improved patient care and safety in its presence. As a leader and seasoned simulation advocate, hospitals will look toward the Ob/Gyn Hospitalist to champion simulation training at their institution.

DISCLOSURE

The authors have no conflicts of interest to disclose.

REFERENCES

1. ACOG Committee Opinion No. 657: The obstetric and gynecology hospitalist. Obstet Gynecol 2016;127:81–5.
2. ACOG Committee Opinion No. 590: Preparing for Clinical Emergencies in Obstetrics and Gynecology. Obstet Gynecol 2014;123(3):722–5.
3. McCue B, Fagnant R, Townsend A, et al. Definitions of obstetric and gynecology hospitalists. Obstet Gynecol 2016;127(2):393–7.
4. Petersen EE, Davis NL, Goodman D, et al. Vital signs: pregnancy-related deaths, United States, 2011–2015, and strategies for prevention, 13 States, 2013–2017. MMWR Morb Mortal Wkly Rep 2019;68:423–9.
5. Draycott T, Sibanda T, Owen L, et al. Does training in obstetric emergencies improve neonatal outcome? BJOG 2005;113(2):177–82.
6. Nestel D, Kelly M, Jolly B, et al. Healthcare simulation education: evidence, theory and practice. West Sussex, UK: Wiley Blackwell; 2018.
7. Institute of Medicine. To err is human: building a safer health system. Washington DC: National Academy Press; 1999.
8. Palaganas J, et al. Defining excellence in simulation programs. Wolters Kluwer; 2015.
9. Eppich W, Cheng A. Promoting Excellence and Reflective Learning in Simulation (PEARLS). Simulat Healthc J Soc Med Simulat 2015;10:106–55.
10. Duff J, Morse KJ, Seelandt J, et al. Debriefing Methods for Simulation in Healthcare: A Systematic Review. Simulat Healthc J Soc Med Simulat 2024;19(1S): S112–21.
11. Dieckmann P, Gaba D, Rall M. Deepening the theoretical foundations of patient simulation as social practice. Simulat Healthc J Soc Med Simulat 2007;2(3): 183–93.
12. American Board of Obstetrics & Gynecology portal, Available at: www.abog.org/maintenance-of-certification/moc—four-parts/improvement-in-medical-practice/practice-improvement-activity-options#Content_C249_Col00, 2024. Accessed November 16, 2023.
13. The Core Competencies for OB and OB/GYN Hospitalists, Society of Ob/Gyn Hospitalists, Available at: http://societyofobgynhospitalists.org, 2022. Accessed November 16, 2023.
14. The Joint Commission. R3 report: Requirement, Rationale, Reference: Provision of care, treatment, and services standards for maternal safety. R3 report issue 24: PC standards for maternal safety. Available at: https://www.jointcommission.org/standards/r3-report/r3-report-issue-24-pc-standards-for-maternal-safety. [Accessed 21 August 2019].
15. ACOG Committee Opinion No, American College of Obstetricians and Gynecologists' Committee on Obstetric Practice. 657: The obstetric and gynecology hospitalist. Obstet Gynecol 2016;127:81–5.
16. Robertson B, Schumacher L, Gosman G, et al. Simulation-based crisis team training for multidisciplinary obstetric providers. Simulat Healthc J Soc Med Simulat 2009;4(2):77–83.

17. Shields A, Vidosh J, Kavanagh L, et al, editors. Obstetric life support manual. Boca Raton, FL: CRC Press; 2024.
18. Fransen AF, van de Ven J, Banga FR, et al. Multi-professional simulation-based team training in obstetric emergencies for improving patient outcomes and trainees' performance. Cochrane Database Syst Rev 2020;12(12):Cd011545.
19. Gupta M, Greene N, Kilpatrick SJ. Timely treatment of severe maternal hypertension and reduction in severe maternal morbidity. Hypertens Pregnancy 2018; 14:55–8.
20. Skupski DW, Lowenwirt IP, Weinbaum FI, et al. Improving hospital systems for the care of women with major obstetric hemorrhage. Obstet Gynecol 2006;107(5): 977–83.

Crisis Management by Obstetrics and Gynecologist Hospitalists: Lessons Learned in a Pandemic

Sarah L. Bradley, MD[a],*, Kim M. Puterbaugh, MD[b]

KEYWORDS

• Obstetrics • Gynecology • Hospitalists • Pandemic • COVID-19 • Leadership

KEY POINTS

- Obstetrics and gynecology (OB/GYN) hospitalists became experts in the care of pregnant patients with COVID-19 disease during the pandemic and collaborated in multidisciplinary teams to optimize patient care outcomes.
- Inpatient OB/GYN care was modified during the pandemic to decrease the risk of virus transmission.
- There are many tools that can be used by OB/GYN hospitalists and hospital systems to improve provider well-being during times of crisis.
- OB/GYN hospitalists served as leaders during the COVID-19 pandemic, advocating for the needs of their patients and their teams.

INTRODUCTION

Four years into the COVID-19 pandemic, its impact continues to reverberate in the medical community. Obstetrics and gynecology (OB/GYN) hospitalists are now well-versed in aspects of COVID-19 management specific to obstetric and gynecologic care.

Pregnancy was determined to be a risk factor for severe disease, leading to an increase in the likelihood of intensive care unit (ICU) admission and death as compared to nonpregnant individuals.[1,2] COVID-19 in pregnancy is also associated with increased risk for adverse perinatal outcomes, such as preeclampsia, preterm birth, and fetal demise.[1] Clinical reviews and practice guidelines summarizing the physiology, clinical course, and management of COVID-19 in pregnancy are now

[a] UW Health Northern Illinois, 1401 East State Street, Rockford, IL 61104, USA; [b] SSM Health / Saint Anthony Hospital, 1000 North Lee Avenue, Suite 1980, Oklahoma City, OK 73102, USA
* Corresponding author.
E-mail address: sbradley@uwhealth.org

Obstet Gynecol Clin N Am 51 (2024) 527–538
https://doi.org/10.1016/j.ogc.2024.04.003
0889-8545/24/© 2024 Elsevier Inc. All rights reserved.

obgyn.theclinics.com

available.[1,2] Recommendations for vaccination to minimize disease spread and severity, including guidance on vaccination in pregnancy, have also been published.[1,3]

OB/GYN hospitalists occupied a unique position during the pandemic as frontline staff. While the medicine, critical care, and emergency service teams were overwhelmed in the early days of the pandemic, other specialties experienced the cancellation of elective visits and procedures, effectively creating a furlough from practice. The need for pregnancy and emergency gynecologic care continued, compelling OB/GYN hospitalist teams to quickly adapt to the changing practice environment.

The need for OB/GYN hospitalist care will likely remain constant or increase with global or national crises in the future. Some predict that pandemic disease will become more frequent,[4] and we know the physiologic changes of pregnancy increase the risk of adverse outcomes from respiratory disease.[5]

With COVID-19 now largely in the rearview mirror, it is vital that we critically assess practice modifications in OB/GYN hospital medicine, to learn which changes best optimized care delivery during the pandemic. Here, we discuss lessons learned from the COVID-19 pandemic through an OB/GYN hospitalist lens, with a focus on clinical care considerations, workforce changes, communication and collaboration, and provider wellness. We end with a discussion on the role of OB/GYN hospitalists as leaders. Our goal is to share what worked well for hospital systems and OB/GYN hospitalist teams during COVID-19, along with a road map of points to consider for future national emergencies.

PATIENT CARE DURING COVID-19

For health care systems during the early days of COVID-19, an overarching goal was to slow the spread of disease while maintaining quality of care. For OB/GYN hospitalist teams, one approach to flattening the curve was to reduce hospitalizations for OB/GYN care. When hospitalization was necessary, other clinical workflow changes were designed to minimize the risk of exposure for both staff and patients. Here, we discuss a number of the strategies employed by OB/GYN hospital teams to achieve these goals.

Reducing Hospitalizations for Obstetrics and Gynecology Care

Keeping people out of the hospital is a key strategy during any pandemic. Minimizing hospitalizations and decreasing hospital length of stay can slow the spread of disease by preventing transmission within the hospital between patients and between staff and patients. Limiting elective hospital care also has the potential to free up space, supplies, and staff. Hospital rooms and operating rooms (ORs) that would normally be used for elective procedures can be redesignated for other use. In many hospital units and for some specialties, both nursing and provider staff can also be redeployed to other units as needed.

OB/GYN hospitalists have a unique and specialized skill set that does not necessarily lend itself to this type of redeployment. However, limiting elective inpatient OB/GYN care can free up the OB/GYN hospitalist team as a means of ensuring adequate backup coverage is available when individual team members are unable to work because of illness. Here, we describe several strategies used by OB/GYN hospitalist teams and departments during COVID-19 to minimize hospitalization for OB/GYN care.

Strategy 1: promote outpatient evaluation and management

A common clinical issue during the early days of the pandemic was how to determine which pregnant patients with COVID-19 disease needed to be evaluated in person or admitted for inpatient care rather than continuing with outpatient management. Algorithms with guidance for making this determination were developed.[6,7] OB/GYN hospitalist teams played an active role in taking such clinical guidance and adapting it for use locally, taking into account the resources and personnel available at their institution. When appropriate, patients with mild disease could be managed at home rather than being evaluated in person in an OB triage or obstetric emergency department (OB-ED) unit.

For common antepartum and postpartum complications of pregnancy, typical care can be modified to reduce hospitalizations. Outpatient management of preterm prelabor rupture of membranes has been described and was instituted at some hospitals.[8,9] For patients at risk of postpartum preeclampsia, telehealth with home blood pressure monitoring decreases hospital readmission.[10] A recently suggested algorithm for management of postpartum preeclampsia may also reduce the need for hospital admission.[11]

Strategy 2: reduce gynecologic surgery volume

During the early days of the pandemic, most hospital systems canceled all elective surgeries, including many gynecologic procedures. For the OB/GYN hospitalist, typically any gynecologic surgeries performed are emergent rather than elective, such as those for ectopic pregnancy or ovarian torsion. In some cases though, surgical management may be optional. For example, an early ectopic pregnancy could be managed with methotrexate rather than surgery, and a missed spontaneous abortion could be appropriately managed with medication or expectantly rather than with dilation and curettage (D&C). Laparoscopy for ectopic pregnancy and D&C for missed abortion should never be considered elective. However, for a hospital system overwhelmed in a pandemic, it may be reasonable to steer patients toward nonsurgical management when such an option exists.[9] Such counseling should continue to emphasize shared decision-making and consider the risks of emergent surgery if outpatient management fails.

Strategy 3: decrease the length of labor admissions

The total time between admission to the labor and delivery (L&D) unit until delivery of the baby is highly variable between patients. Reducing the length of the labor process can decrease the overall amount of time patients spend in the hospital. During the COVID-19 pandemic, these measures included cancellation of elective labor inductions and use of outpatient cervical ripening.[7,9]

Strategy 4: expedite hospital discharge

Early hospital discharge can be facilitated safely for both gynecologic and obstetric patients and was a strategy employed by many OB/GYN hospitalist teams during COVID-19. For gynecologic surgery and c-sections, enhanced recovery after surgery pathways can be implemented to hasten postoperative patient recovery and discharge.[9] For routine postpartum care, many institutions reduced the length of stay for patients after both vaginal deliveries and c-sections.[7,9,12]

Minimizing Risk on Labor and Delivery

OB/GYN hospitalist teams throughout the country provided care to laboring patients with symptomatic COVID-19 disease. In addition, pregnant patients admitted for routine obstetric care were noted to have high rates of asymptomatic severe acute respiratory syndrome coronavirus 2 (SARS-CoV-2) infection early in the pandemic.[13] Many organizations made adjustments to usual care in order to decrease transmission risk.

The availability of personal protective equipment (PPE) was a critical concern early in the pandemic.[13,14] Institutions developed guidelines for PPE use for both routine obstetric and gynecologic care and patients with suspected or known COVID-19 on OB/GYN units. The likelihood of aerosolization of SARS-Co-V-2 particles during the second stage of labor and whether N95 masks were required became particularly controversial.[13] Although based on recommendations from the Centers for Disease Control and state public health departments, guidelines for PPE use varied widely between institutions.

The goal of physically cohorting patients with suspected or known COVID led some organizations to designate a COVID OR. For one of the authors, the COVID OR was located within the main OR unit approximately 7 minutes away from L&D. Staff education was provided and simulations were performed so the team was prepared to perform cesarean sections in the new location. A lower threshold for recommending cesarean section was suggested to minimize the chance of emergent cesarean for fetal bradycardia. As emergently performed caesarean deliveries are more likely to require patient intubation and may increase the chance of staff donning PPE incorrectly, considering a lowered threshold for surgical delivery made sense in these circumstances.

As the pandemic went on, procedures were developed to disinfect OR and patient rooms recently vacated by patients with COVID disease. These procedures required up to several hours, depending on room size and air flow exchange. However, taking an OR or patient room out of service for this length of time could create critical space shortages. In their role as patient safety officer, OB/GYN hospitalists worked with nursing staff in these situations to actively manage the L&D unit to optimize patient care.

THE PANDEMIC WORKFORCE

OB/GYN departments and hospitalist teams needed to quickly adapt to the changing practice environment in the beginning of the COVID-19 pandemic. Anecdotally, the authors are aware of several different types of staffing modifications that occurred throughout the country including in our own institutions. Planning for workforce adaptation during a pandemic includes several key considerations, but can be thought of in two main categories. First, there is a need for flexibility in the type of work performed by individual providers to meet the change in clinical needs. Second, contingency plans need to account for the likelihood that providers will become ill and unable to work.

There was a huge shift toward telephone and video visits in outpatient OB/GYN clinics, as previous barriers related to billing for telehealth visits were reduced or eliminated early in the pandemic. The overall number of clinic visits was also significantly limited, such that some providers were able to shift to inpatient work. Creating clearly defined responsibilities for each inpatient clinical role was helpful for teams in which clinicians were deployed outside of their typical job.

In the hospital, some OB/GYN hospitalist groups and departments initially divided providers into COVID and non-COVID teams.[7] The COVID cohort of providers took on the care of patients with COVID disease and the non-COVID team did not. When contemplating this type of strategy, OB/GYN hospitalist teams should consider the risk factors for individual providers. It was suggested those at particularly high risk should be offered low-risk work responsibilities or a leave of absence.[7] Economic incentives (ie, hazard pay) could be offered by health care systems considering this type of strategy; however, those providers choosing not to practice outside of their scope should not be penalized.[15]

At some hospitals, the OB/GYN hospitalist shift schedule was altered to include longer shifts or shifts clustered closer together in time than usual. These team cohorts and schedule changes were intended to limit potential exposures to fewer providers in a given time period, while keeping other providers in reserve. The providers in reserve were expected to observe social distancing guidelines while away from work to limit exposure risk, thus decreasing the chance of becoming ill themselves.

Hospital systems early in the pandemic also grappled with the question of whether providers with high-risk exposure to COVID-19 should continue to work. In some instances, health care workers with high-risk exposures continued work because of staffing shortages.[13]

COLLABORATION AND COMMUNICATION DURING COVID-19

During the COVID-19 pandemic, most hospitals instituted an incident command system or similar emergency management structure to coordinate efforts. General principles and a framework for emergency management responses can be found elsewhere[16] and can be reviewed with an eye toward OB/GYN hospitalist team pandemic preparedness.

The best communication strategy will depend on the needs and resources of each specific institution; however, all systems should have a leadership chain of command clearly identified. The incident command team is responsible for directing the efforts of supply chain, laboratory, pharmacy, security, environmental services, and information technology as well as facilitating communication between those teams and clinical staff. The incident command team should function as the one designated leadership communication source and should include representation from all clinical departments.[7]

From the OB/GYN hospitalist team, there should be a designated leader in direct and frequent formal communication with incident command who can advocate for the specific needs of pregnant patients and OB/GYN staff. Early in the COVID-19 pandemic, OB/GYN hospitalists pushed for appropriate PPE for hospital staff. The receptiveness of system leadership to hearing these types of suggestions and concerns was crucial to the staff on the front lines. As stated by a member of the Society of OB/GYN Hospitalists (SOGH) when surveyed about went well during the early days of the COVID-19 pandemic, "Our hospital has a COVID team. They have been very receptive to testing and proper PPE use."[14]

The OB/GYN hospitalist team also needed to collaborate and communicate directly with OB/GYN department and nursing leadership during the pandemic. These three groups should work together to develop new workflows and policies impacting OB/GYN hospital units, as any change is likely to have an impact on each of their respective teams. During COVID-19, some systems reported use of daily physician/nursing leadership huddles.[17] For any emergent change in guidance, these teams should utilize a preplanned notification system.[16]

Within the OB/GYN hospitalist team, the designated leader should develop a communication plan for acquisition and delivery of new information to team members. With the overwhelming volume of new clinical information during the pandemic, some OB/GYN hospitalist teams appointed a single member with fewer clinical responsibilities to keep abreast of current recommendations, while others looked to their maternal–fetal medicine (MFM) colleagues to summarize latest clinical updates. As operational workflows changed rapidly as well, there was a need for thoughtful consideration as to the frequency and mode of communication for both clinical and operations updates. A medical hospitalist team reported success with a nightly email sent to clinicians as well as twice weekly virtual town halls.[17] One OB/GYN team noted an increase in staff member confidence with regular unit-based updates with Q&A sessions.[18] A member of SOGH reported, "I am proud of the leadership providing education, training, and daily updates," as an example of what worked well during the early pandemic.[14] An illustration showing these communication pathways is shown in **Fig. 1**.

Collaboration Within the Health Care System

The incident command system and communication pathways as described in the preceding section can facilitate cooperation between the OB/GYN hospitalist team and other units and teams within the health care system. During the COVID-19 pandemic, OB/GYN hospitalists needed to collaborate more than ever before with emergency services, general medicine, and critical care teams. Specialty specific input is important to optimize care for OB/GYN patients at the time of initial presentation, when making decisions about admission, and during hospitalization. As to the setting of initial evaluation, most hospital systems have an established workflow designating the appropriate unit for a patient presenting with an OB/GYN concern or nonrelated concern during pregnancy, which may be the emergency department, OB triage, or a specialty OB-ED. These established workflows were sometimes modified during COVID, such that patients presenting with symptoms of illness were placed into a physically separated cohort. When deciding whether an ill patient requires hospitalization, nonobstetricians performing the initial evaluation benefited from OB/GYN hospitalist guidance as to how admission criteria may differ in the pregnant population.

For pregnant patients after viability, decisions made as to which unit is most appropriate for the initial evaluation and for hospitalization need to account for fetal monitoring, as this is a vital sign for pregnant patients.[1,13] In some institutions, pregnant

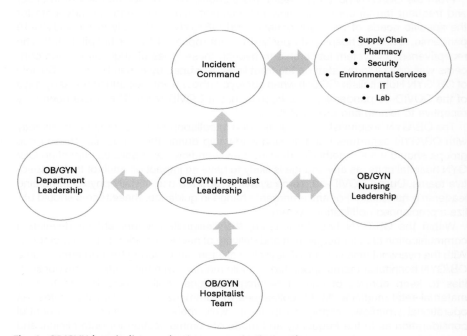

Fig. 1. OB/GYN hospitalist pandemic communication pathways.

patients mildly ill with COVID were managed on the L&D floor to easily accommodate the need for fetal monitoring. Some systems noted that these patients were kept in negative pressure rooms if possible; or if not, they were placed in a physical cohort away from other pregnant patients.[13,18] At other institutions, pregnant patients with mild to moderate COVID were placed on general medical floors. Critically ill pregnant patients are typically managed in the ICU; however, at least one system retrofitted L&D rooms with ICU monitoring capabilities to accommodate critically ill COVID patients on L&D.[18] For patients placed on general medical floors and in the ICU, unless remote fetal monitoring was possible, nursing staff were needed to perform in-person fetal monitoring. One drawback of in-person fetal monitoring away from the L&D floor is that it takes away from the nursing pool available on L&D. Another disadvantage during a pandemic is that it leads to an increase in interaction and potential exposure to pandemic illness between the L&D and general medical or ICU staff. The ability to perform remote fetal monitoring would clearly have alleviated some of the logistical challenges that arose when caring for pregnant patients in the ED, general medical floors, and in the ICU during COVID-19. We recommend that when planning for future expansion or renovation of these areas, hospital systems should solicit input from the OB/GYN hospitalist team and any other patient care teams that may have specialized care needs.

For pregnant patients hospitalized with moderate to critical COVID during the pandemic, OB/GYN hospitalist teams played an invaluable role by collaborating with their colleagues on the medicine hospitalist, infectious disease, and critical care teams. Obstetric-specific guidance was needed for these patients regarding the appropriate unit for care, steroid use, proning, maternal oxygen saturation requirement for fetal oxygenation, delivery timing, and mode of delivery. At some institutions, the MFM team may have been primarily responsible for providing these recommendations. For other systems, these management decisions were collaboration between the OB/GYN hospitalist and MFM teams or came from the OB/GYN hospitalist team alone for institutions without a high-risk obstetrics consultant available. A multidisciplinary team-based approach is a foundational element of OB/GYN hospitalist medicine, and this was clearly demonstrated during the pandemic.

Regional Care Coordination

General guidance for regional coordination in the setting of a pandemic or disaster has been described previously.[16] Purchasing and stockpiling of supplies, equipment, and pharmaceuticals can be coordinated either regionally or at the state level.[16] For OB/GYN hospitalist medicine, regional coordination may be helpful in the setting of supply chain issues and shortages of specific medications such as oxytocin and other uterotonics.

A unique consideration that arose during the COVID-19 pandemic for one of the authors was determining the appropriate unit to care for a critically ill pregnant teenager. Adult critical care specialists may be reluctant to care for a pregnant pediatric patient; however, in the absence of a local pediatric ICU (PICU) or OB-specific ICU, this may be the best option. Alternatively, regional collaboration can identify availability of PICU beds and develop plans for transfer when appropriate. Maternity bed space including critical care beds and general L&D, antepartum, and postpartum beds could be tracked in real time. Regional collaboration could also support care for pregnant patients at non-maternity hospitals through the use of telemedicine and remote consults.

During the COVID-19 pandemic, regions throughout the country worked together to coordinate distribution of clinical information. One large system reported the development of a disaster manual and regional communication plan for obstetric hospitals.[18]

Illinois utilized its state perinatal quality collaborative to host weekly statewide webinars to provide clinical updates during the pandemic.[19] Regional coordination based on identification of maternal levels of care has been suggested by the American College of Obstetricians and Gynecologists (ACOG),[20] and many states have already instituted neonatal levels of care. This type of coordination should be encouraged to facilitate information sharing and best outcomes for patients.

PROVIDER WELLNESS DURING COVID-19

The toll the pandemic took on physicians and specifically OB/GYN hospitalists is still not fully recognized or understood. The challenges at work were many, beginning with fears about personal health risk. Initially, we were uncertain how effective PPE would be in preventing transmission of the virus. In many cases, we had inadequate PPE supplies and needed to reuse face masks and N95 respirators for days or even weeks at a time. At some institutions, physicians were told they could not use their own personal respirators for concern this would scare nursing staff and patients. Fears about personal health risk were not unfounded, as several OB/GYN physicians died from COVID-19,[21] including a 2nd year OB/GYN resident working in Texas.[22]

At the onset of the COVID-19 crisis, the immediate concern for health care systems was the surge of patients ill with COVID presenting to the ED and in need of ICU care. This response was appropriate and vital, and hospital administrators needed to make critical decisions about distribution of limited resources. However, the lack of prioritization of PPE on OB/GYN units contributed to the moral injury felt by some OB/GYN hospitalists and put the health and lives of patients and providers at risk.

The unknown science was particularly challenging in the beginning of the pandemic. There were no tests for SARS-CoV-2 in the beginning, let alone guidelines for management during pregnancy. Those in the OB/GYN hospitalist community suspected that pregnancy would increase the risk for morbidity and mortality related to COVID based on our prior experience with influenza and other respiratory viruses.

Conflicting information contributed to medical distrust among the public which made our jobs harder. As physicians, OB/GYN hospitalists are likely more comfortable than the layperson with evolving scientific information and changing guidelines; however, the accelerated pace of new information was dizzying. In the first weeks of the pandemic, daily press briefings from the White House, state and local officials, and hospital administrators with rapidly changing and conflicting recommendations became overwhelming. Public confusion led to an escalating erosion of trust in the medical community.

Some patients refused mask and social distancing mandates, putting not just themselves but hospital staff at risk. Attempting to educate patients with fixed beliefs based on false information took its toll on OB/GYN hospitalists. We work in a fast-paced specialty where timely decisions save lives, and the added time and energy we spent on COVID education was exhausting and often felt futile.

The professional stressors experienced by OB/GYN hospitalists during the pandemic were compounded by challenges at home. Many had fears about bringing COVID home from work and infecting loved ones, particularly medically vulnerable family members. Some OB/GYN hospitalists practiced elaborate disinfection routines or even isolated within their homes or moved out to prevent transmission of the virus to their family.

As schools and daycares shut down, many OB/GYN hospitalists needed to navigate alternative options for schooling for their children. With minimal childcare options available, some needed to take a leave of absence to care for young children. Marriages and partnerships felt the strain of lost income as many nonessential workers were furloughed during stay-at-home orders. The loss of shared social activities and in some cases, forced togetherness because of working from home, were also a source of stress.

Wellness Strategies for Providers

We had to find ways to cope with the intense stress at work and home during the pandemic. The SOGH hosted a webinar[23] to discuss effective strategies to improve wellness, including the recommendations listed in **Fig. 2**. The added stress and uncertainty of the pandemic made sleep both more vital and elusive for many OB/GYN hospitalists. Scrolling through COVID case numbers, articles, and work emails at night made falling asleep more difficult. Adhering to good sleep hygiene—turning off screens half an hour before bed, creating/maintaining an uncluttered, dark, quiet space to sleep, using sleep apps, and allowing for an adequate amount of sleep—all became critical to facing the following days' challenges. With gyms and indoor exercise classes closed, outdoor and home exercise became the healthiest option during the pandemic. Cooking at home became more common during lock down, with eating out and ordering in both less safe and sometimes unavailable. Focusing on healthy meals (not just comfort food such as bread and desserts) was challenging but a better long-term health strategy. Connecting with family and friends through newer technologies such as Zoom calls lessened social isolation. Conversations from across the street and drive-by celebrations replaced in-person parties. Many families spent time with pets as a safe and comforting connection, which lowers blood pressure and increases wellness.

The levels of anxiety and depression OB/GYN hospitalists experienced varied from frustrating to clinically significant. Focusing on basic healthy habits, such as sleep and exercise, was critical. Finding support from peers experiencing similar challenges, such as through the SOGH's Team Thrive, helped. For those with symptoms severe enough to impair their ability to function at home and work, medications and therapy were important but sometimes difficult to access during the pandemic.

Wellness Strategies for Health Care Systems

Our work as OB/GYN hospitalists did not pause during the height of the pandemic and for many has continued at the same pace, leaving little time to reflect. Many staff retired, especially older, more experienced nurses and physicians. This makes staffing L&D units harder now, requiring those still employed to work more shifts. There are wellness strategies health care systems could deploy that may help with employee retention.

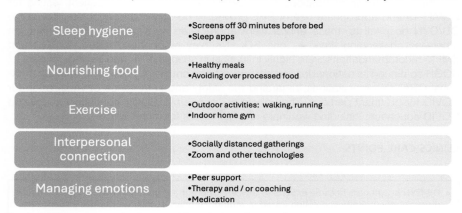

Fig. 2. Wellness strategies for providers during the pandemic.

First, barriers to mental health counseling, including scheduling and stigma, could be lowered by making counseling opt-out to help OB/GYN hospitalists process the trauma they experienced during the pandemic. Increasing mental health resources, particularly during off-hours, such as through online counseling, will be vital going forward. Post-pandemic support groups are also a valuable resource for professionals. SOGH has hosted quarterly wellness seminars,[24] where members share the challenges we faced during the pandemic. Finally, allowing more time away from work duties for those staff who worked throughout the pandemic would provide time and space for recovery. Hospitals should consider funding locums or other staffing options for 1 to 2 months of sabbatical. Postpandemic sabbaticals could be rotated to be less disruptive than furloughing multiple physicians at once. This strategy incurs significant cost; however, in the long run, it may decrease costs via increased retention of experienced staff members who may otherwise be lost to burnout and early retirement.

OBSTETRICS AND GYNECOLOGY HOSPITALISTS AS LEADERS

OB/GYN hospitalists serve as leaders in our units, hospitals, and nationally, advocating for our patients and our team. During the COVID-19 crisis, the skills we routinely utilize were critical to managing the crisis. We assessed how to best manage patients with potential or confirmed COVID in our specific settings, to both provide them optimal care and to prevent the spread of the virus to others. We identified needs, proposed solutions, and ran simulations to determine whether our plans would work.

OB/GYN hospitalists also did what leaders must do in any crisis: we disseminated information as it became available, dispelled rumors, identified staff who were struggling, and improved morale to the best of our ability. We adjusted staffing schedules to limit physician exposure to the virus and then again as staff became ill.

We determined the role of learners, such as residents, on our teams. We had to balance our residents' need to continue their education with our duty to keep them safe. OB/GYN hospitalists advocated for our patients, our nurses, our housekeeping staff, and ourselves with hospital administration. We requested appropriate supplies of PPE. We coordinated between units, especially the ICU, when pregnant women with COVID became critically ill.

Despite the absence of peer-reviewed data on COVID in pregnancy, we needed to act. The SOGH, as nationally elected leadership in our field, pooled our knowledge and developed consensus guidelines. Our first position statement was released on April 10, 2020. The recommendations for universal masking, universal patient testing for COVID-19 and appropriate use of PPE proved to be sound and accurate. For some OB/GYN hospitalists, these efforts were appreciated as a positive event during an otherwise challenging time. As one SOGH survey respondent stated, "SOGH and SMFM recommendations were highly influential in shaping PPE and testing policies."[14] SOGH continued its national leadership role, signing onto joint statements with other national OB/GYN organizations, regarding the safety and importance of vaccination for COVID for pregnant persons. Throughout the pandemic, SOGH continued to develop COVID education, including webinars and guidelines for members.[23]

CLINICS CARE POINTS

- OB/GYN hospitalists became experts in the care of pregnant patients with COVID-19 disease during the pandemic and collaborated in multidisciplinary teams to optimize patient care outcomes.

- Inpatient OB/GYN care was modified during the pandemic to decrease the risk of virus transmission.
- There are many tools that can be used by OB/GYN hospitalists and hospital systems to improve provider well-being during times of crisis.
- OB/GYN hospitalists served as leaders during the COVID-19 pandemic, advocating for the needs of their patients and their teams.

SUMMARY

Four years after the declaration of a worldwide pandemic, it is difficult to fully recall the fear and disruption initially caused by COVID-19. As OB/GYN hospitalists, we made life-altering decisions for our patients, our staff, ourselves and our families with limited scientific data, rapidly changing guidelines, and inconsistently available PPE. Births and gynecologic emergencies did not pause for the pandemic. As we reflect on lessons learned during the pandemic, the role of OB/GYN hospitalists as leaders is clear. Our expertise is vital, and we must continue to advocate for our patients and ourselves. OB/GYN hospitalists need to be a part of hospital and national leadership, so we can participate in critical decision-making when the next crisis occurs.

DISCLOSURE

The authors have no financial disclosures to report. Dr. K.M. Puterbaugh has previously served as the president of the Society of OB/GYN Hospitalists.

REFERENCES

1. Jamieson DJ, Rasmussen SA. An update on COVID-19 and pregnancy. Am J Obstet Gynecol 2022;226(2):177–86.
2. Nana M, Hodson K, Lucas N, et al. Diagnosis and management of Covid-19 in pregnancy. BMJ 2022;377:e069739.
3. Society for Maternal-Fetal Medicine. COVID-19 vaccination in pregnancy. 2023. Available at: https://s3.amazonaws.com/cdn.smfm.org/media/4181/SMFM_COVID_Vaccine_2023.pdf. [Accessed 4 January 2024].
4. Marani M, Katul GG, Pan WK, et al. Intensity and frequency of extreme novel epidemics. Proc Natl Acad Sci USA 2021;118(35). https://doi.org/10.1073/pnas.2105482118.
5. Stone S, Nelson-Piercy C. Respiratory disease in pregnancy. Obstet Gynaecol Reprod Med 2007 May;17(5):140–6.
6. American College of Obstetricians and Gynecologists and Society for Maternal-Fetal Medicine. Outpatient assessment and management for pregnant women with suspected or confirmed novel coronavirus (COVID-19). Available at: COVID-19-Algorithm.pdf (physiciansweekly.com). Accessed May 17, 2024.
7. Gold S, Clarfield L, Johnstone J, et al. Adapting obstetric and neonatal services during the COVID-19 pandemic: a scoping review. BMC Pregnancy Childbirth 2022;22(1):119.
8. Chacon KM, Bryant M, Allison S, et al. Outpatient Expectant Management of Premature Rupture of Membranes for Women Who Decline Augmentation [14F]. Obstet Gynecol 2019;133:65S–6S.
9. Duzyj CM, Thornburg LL, Han CS. Practice modification for pandemics: a model for surge planning in obstetrics. Obstet Gynecol 2020;136(2):237–51.

10. Hoppe KK, Thomas N, Zernick M, et al. Telehealth with remote blood pressure monitoring compared with standard care for postpartum hypertension. Am J Obstet Gynecol 2020;223(4):585–8.
11. Cagino K, Prabhu M, Sibai B. Is magnesium sulfate therapy warranted in all cases of late postpartum severe hypertension? A suggested approach to a clinical conundrum. Am J Obstet Gynecol 2023;229(6):641–6.
12. Bornstein E, Gulersen M, Husk G, et al. Early postpartum discharge during the COVID-19 pandemic. J Perinat Med 2020;48(9):1008–12.
13. Dayal AK, Razavi AS, Jaffer AK, et al. COVID-19 in obstetrics 2020: the experience at a New York City medical center. J Perinat Med 2020;48(9):892–9.
14. Society of OB/GYN Hospitalists. The OB/GYN Hospitalist Experience During Coronavirus Disease 2019 (COVID-19). Education and COVID-19 Resources. Available at: https://h5740a.a2cdn1.secureserver.net/wp-content/uploads/2021/05/SOGH_COVID_SURVEY_FINALforwebsite.pdf. [Accessed 2 January 2024].
15. Ethical considerations for the delivery of obstetric and gynecologic care during a pandemic. committee statement no. 6. american college of obstetricians and gynecologists. Obstet Gynecol 2023;142:225–30.
16. Einav S, Hick JL, Hanfling D, et al, Task Force for Mass Critical Care; Task Force for Mass Critical Care, Task Force for Mass Critical Care. Surge capacity logistics: care of the critically ill and injured during pandemics and disasters: CHEST consensus statement. Chest 2014;146(4 Suppl):e17S–43S.
17. Bowden K, Burnham EL, Keniston A, et al. Harnessing the Power of Hospitalists in Operational Disaster Planning: COVID-19. J Gen Intern Med 2020;35(9):2732–7.
18. Harvey S, Zalud I. Obstetric hospital preparedness for a pandemic: an obstetrical critical care perspective in response to COVID-19. J Perinat Med 2020;48(9):874–82.
19. Illinois Perinatal Quality Collaborative. Covid-19 information for ILPQC hospital teams. Available at: https://ilpqc.org/covid-19-information/. [Accessed 26 January 2024].
20. American College of Obstetricians and Gynecologists and Society for Maternal–Fetal Medicine, Menard MK, Kilpatrick S, Saade G, et al. Levels of maternal care. Am J Obstet Gynecol 2015;212(3):259–71.
21. Hoenig LJ. In memoriam: Physicians who have died of COVID-19 in the United States. Clin Dermatol 2020 November-December;38(6):771–2.
22. Gallman S. 28-year-old Houston doctor dies after battle with coronavirus, family says. CNN; 2020. Available at: https://www.cnn.com/2020/09/22/us/houston-adeline-fagan-covid-19-death/index.html. [Accessed 31 January 2024].
23. COVID-19 resources. Society of OB/GYN Hospitalists. Available at: https://societyofobgynhospitalists.org/portfolio/covid-19-education-and-resources/. [Accessed 31 January 2024].
24. SOGH Team Thrive Wellness and Peer Support. Society of OB/GYN Hospitalists. Available at: https://societyofobgynhospitalists.org/portfolio/thrive/. [Accessed 31 January 2024].

Diversity, Equity, and Inclusion

Obstetrics and Gynecologist Hospitalists' Impact on Maternal Mortality

Julianne DeMartino, MD[a],*, Monique Yoder Katsuki, MD[b],
Megan R. Ansbro, MD, PhD[b]

KEYWORDS

- Maternal morbidity and mortality • Trauma informed care
- Obstetrics and gynecology hospitalist • Diversity • equity and inclusion

KEY POINTS

- Understanding maternal morbidity and mortality (M&M) trends.
- Reducing preventable causes of morbidity and mortality (M&M).
- Promotion of patient agency with shared decision-making and trauma-informed care.
- Champions for diversity, equity, and inclusion education with recognition of disparities in health care.
- Creating seamless transitions between hospital-based care and community-based services.

Statement regarding inclusivity and language: We would like to acknowledge the importance of recognizing and affirming the diverse identities and experiences of individuals receiving obstetric and gynecologic care. While historically, discussions in the field of Obstetrics & Gynecology have often centered on terms like 'women' and 'mothers,' we want to emphasize that our understanding and language have evolved to be more inclusive. We acknowledge that not all individuals who may receive obstetric and gynecologic care identify strictly within these categories, and while historical terminology may be referenced, we strive to use inclusive language and terminology in our original content and wish to promote normalizing this practice in our field.

INTRODUCTION

In March of 2023, the maternal mortality rate in the United States (US) once again became the focus of public attention. The data from the National Center for Health

[a] University Hospitals MacDonald Women's Hospital, 2101 Adelbert Road, Cleveland, OH 44106, USA; [b] Cleveland Clinic Foundation, Obstetric and Gynecologic Institute, 9500 Euclid Avenue/A81, Cleveland, OH 44195, USA
* Corresponding author.
E-mail address: demartj2@ccf.org

Obstet Gynecol Clin N Am 51 (2024) 539–558
https://doi.org/10.1016/j.ogc.2024.05.007   **obgyn.theclinics.com**
0889-8545/24/© 2024 Elsevier Inc. All rights are reserved, including those for text and data mining, AI training, and similar technologies.

Statistics demonstrated that the maternal mortality rate increased by 60% between 2019 and 2021 with 754 maternal deaths in 2019 compared to 1205 in 2021.[1] Though a quarter of the deaths were attributed to coronavirus disease 2019 (COVID 19) between 2020 and 2021, this does not detract from the significance of the pre-COVID 19 maternal mortality rate that had doubled between 1999 and 2019.[2–4] While the data demonstrated that the maternal mortality rate increased for all races and ethnicities during 2020 and 2021, the maternal mortality rate during COVID 19 increased disproportionately with 69.9 deaths per 100000 live births for black women, 26.6 deaths per 100000 for white women, and 28 deaths per 100000 in Hispanic women.[1] Additionally, American Indian and Alaska Native women have had the highest increase in the median maternal mortality rate between 1999 and 2019.[3] Race and ethnicity have not been the only factors in the increased maternal mortality rate. Women aged 40 and over have a 6.8 times higher mortality rate than those women under the age of 25.[1]

Despite the increasing maternal mortality rate in the US, the rate of delivery-related in-hospital maternal mortality has declined by 50%. This finding was demonstrated in a large cross-sectional study, *Maternal Mortality and Severe Maternal Morbidity in the United States, 2008 to 2021* by Fink *and colleagues*[4] The study looked at 11 million inpatient discharges between Q1 of 2008 to Q4 of 2021 and found that delivery-related in-hospital maternal mortality rates had significantly decreased for all racial, ethnic, and age groups regardless of their mode of delivery. Conversely, the study demonstrated that the severe maternal morbidity rate had increased and was a contributing factor in the overall increasing maternal mortality rate in the US.[4] Given that the overall maternal mortality rate has increased despite a decrease in the inpatient setting, it is important to identify factors contributing to this discrepancy and create strategies for improvement in maternal health care both in and out of the hospital. The study cites that over the past decade, national initiatives to heighten the safety and quality of patient-care with evidence-based standards of practice and the awareness of disparities in health care are contributing to the decline in the inpatient mortality rate.[4] National initiatives such as patient safety bundles, evidence-based protocols and toolkits, checklists, simulations, and the growing presence of the obstetrics and gynecology (OB/GYN) hospitalist on labor and delivery (L&D) units play a crucial role in decreasing inpatient maternal mortality rates. For the intent of this review, the focus will be on the role of the OB/GYN hospitalist who is uniquely positioned to provide timely emergent care for patients on L&D, safe subsequent inpatient-care, and has the ability to facilitate closing the gap between inpatient and outpatient-care. This care is rooted in best practices and innovative strategies, maintaining collaborative relationships with multidisciplinary team members to create seamless high-quality care, identifying common causes of morbidity and mortality (M&M), being knowledgeable with regard to cultural humility in care, and lastly, integrating community though building an understanding of the patient population, values, resources, and creating opportunities for successful care beyond the walls of the hospital.

CLINICAL STRATEGIES TO DECREASE MATERNAL MORTALITY THROUGH THE REDUCTION OF SEVERE MATERNAL MORBIDITY
Evidence-Based Practices and the Obstetrics and Gynecology Hospitalist

Evidence-based practices are valuable tools to address preventable causes of severe morbidities and mortalities, to include but not exclusive to, obstetric hemorrhage, hypertensive crisis, shoulder dystocia, sepsis, mental health, substance use disorder, and inequities in health care.[5–8] The increasing presence of OB/GYN hospitalists on L&D provides an opportunity to be an integral part of utilizing evidence-based practices and champion consistency of patient-care.[9] Evidence-based practices make use of established clinical guidelines to standardize patient-care providing consistency and improve outcomes. This approach moves away from clinical variation in critical tasks during high acuity situations that could be a subject to error due to infrequent management of such events, fatigue, the overall stress of the situation, and caregiver biases. Standardizing evidence-based practices lends itself to ensuring that a diverse patient population will consistently be provided the established standard-of-care. Resources such as practice guidelines, toolkits, and safety bundles are available to create standardized practices, protocols, and checklists and yet gaps in guideline implementation occur. The lack of adherence to guidelines has resulted in 30% to 40% of patients receiving treatment that is not evidence-based and 20% to 25% receive treatments that are either not warranted or harmful.[5] Physician knowledge and attitudes, complexity, and applicability of the established guidelines and organizational constraints were cited as possible barriers to protocol implementation.[6] Strategies to overcome such barriers not only at the physician level, but as an interdisciplinary team, include increasing awareness with dissemination of guidelines, having visual prompts such as posters and providing opportunities for education. Additionally, utilizing physicians, nurses, and interdepartmental collaborators promotes a team approach and enhances adherence to mutually agreed-upon evidence-based protocols. And lastly, creating protocols that are mindful of the organizational infrastructure and resources enhance the success of adherence.[4–6]

Early Recognition of the Decompensating Patient: Maternal Early Warning Triggers

A tool that can be utilized to decrease maternal morbidity is the development of an early warning tool that has set vital signs that can aid in the early identification of a decompensating patient. A large prospective study by Shields *and colleagues*[6] "Use of Maternal Early Warning Trigger Tools Reduces Maternal Morbidity" demonstrated that establishing and utilizing early warning criteria, increased the early recognition of sepsis, hemorrhage, hypertensive emergencies, and cardiopulmonary dysfunction.[6–9] There are multiple studies that have examined the vital sign parameters that are best used in pregnant patients and toolkits are readily available.[6–8] An example of how the early maternal warning signs may be combined with an escalation plan can be seen in **Fig. 1**. This example creates an identification and escalation plan in 1 simplified model. Its intent is to create a situational awareness for the care team as to what maternal warning signs must be acknowledged and what the corresponding escalation of care should entail.

Limiting Interventions During Labor

Limiting intervention during labor and birth has also been shown to improve patient outcomes and satisfaction.[9] Limited intervention strategies include collaborative efforts between the patient, obstetrician-gynecologists, nurses, midwives, and doulas. Educating and creating space for shared decision-making with regard to pain management, comfort options, fetal monitoring, amniotomy and use of medications provides the opportunity for minimal intervention and an understanding of interventions that may be recommended based on clinical indicators.[9]

Preventing the First Cesarean and Optimizing Vaginal Birth

Preventing the first cesarean section is another valuable strategy to improve obstetric outcomes. Between 1996 and 2021, the cesarean rate in the US has increased by 55%.[10] In 2021, 32.2% of live births were cesareans with 3 out of 5 being primary cesareans and 4 out of 5 women who had a primary cesarean will have a repeat in future births.[10] When the 2021 statistics were further analyzed by race and ethnicity, 36.2%

Maternal Early Warning criteria	Action When Criteria Identified
• New Onset Systolic BP ≤90 or ≥140 and/or • New Onset Diastolic BP ≥90	• Criteria in **BLUE BOX** is to be reevaluated in 10 minutes and provider notified of both findings.

• Temperature ≤36° C (96.5 ° F) or ≥38° C (100.4 °F)
• Heart Rate ≤50 or ≥120
• Respiratory Rate ≤10 or ≥30
• Oxygen saturation <95%
• Oliguria: less than 30cc/hr for 2 hours
• Systolic BP ≥ 150 or Diastolic BP ≥ 105
	• Criteria in YELLOW BOX requires a bedside evaluation
	  • If the provider is not immediately available, give verbal report and determine plan of action to include:
	    • Frequency of re-evaluation
	    • Criteria for immediate physician notification
	    • Diagnostic or therapeutic interventions
	    • When will bedside evaluation occur

• Systolic BP ≥ 160 and/or Diastolic BP ≥ 110 • Patient reporting unremitting headache, shortness of breath, agitation, confusion	• Criteria in ORANGE BOX requires immediate bedside evaluation.

Rapid Response – Acute critical changes in a patient's status that requires immediate mobilization of multiple providers.

Fig. 1. Maternal early warning triggers. (*Source:* DeMartino, J, Train the Trainer, Society of OB/GYN Hospitalists.)

of live births for Black women were cesarean deliveries and 30.8% and 31.4% were cesarean deliveries for white and Hispanic women, respectively.[11,12] Cesarean sections have 2.7 times the risk of severe maternal morbidity when compared to vaginal delivery. Patients undergoing a cesarean section have higher rates of hemorrhage, blood transfusions, uterine rupture, hysterectomy, infection, and placenta accreta spectrum in future pregnancies.[13–15] Utilizing established guidelines and toolkits that provide guidance for promoting vaginal birth can be instrumental in lowering the cesarean section rate. Such strategies include protocols for management of fetal malpresentation with occiput posterior in the second stage of labor, external cephalic version and breech extraction of the second twin.[13,14] Other strategies to decrease cesarean deliveries include the development of checklists that define the phases of labor and labor dystocia management.[14] Development of protocols for the identification and management of category II fetal heart tracings and the use of operative vaginal deliveries in appropriate candidates may also lead to decreasing the cesarean section rate.[14,16] When the first cesarean section is medically indicated, patient education and counseling for a trial of labor after cesarean (TOLAC) is another strategy to decrease morbidity from repeat cesarean sections. This counseling should include the risks and benefits of a trial of labor versus a repeat cesarean section and may include the use of the Vaginal Birth After Cesarean Section (VBAC) calculator published by the National Institute of Child Health and Human Development.[17] This calculator was originally developed in 2007 and utilized multiple variables to include race and ethnicity as predictors of the likelihood for a successful TOLAC.[17] More recently, a new VBAC calculator was developed and no longer based outcomes on race and ethnicity as predictors of success. The new VBAC calculator calibration curve was similar to the previous curve in accuracy without the variables of race and ethnicity and therefore determined that the success of a TOLAC using race as a variable is not biologically-based but rather a component of systemic racism, social determinants of health and bias.[5]

Shared Decision-Making & Respectful Care: Optimizing Care Delivery to Optimize Outcomes

Team Birth–In the US, birthing people are more likely to experience mistreatment, severe morbidity, and mortality compared to any other high-income country.[18] These issues are even more likely to occur for people identifying with minoritized populations.[18] Additionally, approximately 84% of maternal deaths are thought to be preventable, and 80% of preventable adverse events are attributable to poor communication.[19,20] To optimize and improve equity in patient experience and health outcomes, systems must implement measures to ensure that patients consistently receive respectful, collaborative, compassionate, and culturally competent care at all times. Numerous initiatives, including Ariadne Labs' TeamBirth and Association of Women's Health, Obstetric and Neonatal Nurses's (AWHONN's) Respectful Maternity Care (RMC) program are currently being implemented across the US and are centered on improving care delivery in order to improve health outcomes and eliminate inequities in outcomes.[21]

TeamBirth is an innovative inpatient obstetric care model designed by Ariadne Labs, a center for health care innovation at Brigham and Women's Hospital and the Harvard T.H. Chan School of Public Health.[21] TeamBirth utilizes a simplified, white board-based team rounding model for obstetric care that centers 4 key principles including: psychologic safety, shared decision-making, equitable care, and closed-loop communication.[21] The model is designed to ensure that inclusive, equitable care is consistently provided for every patient, which improves safety, health outcomes, and patient experience. TeamBirth has now been implemented at over 130 sites across the US and has demonstrated remarkable improvements in clinical outcomes (cesarean section rates), patient experience scores, and reduction in inequities in outcomes for minoritized populations.[21] The materials needed to implement TeamBirth can be accessed at no cost on the Ariadne Labs' website and if desired the team Ariadne Labs will provide implementation support for TeamBirth for a fee depending on a facility's size and needs.[21]

Association of Women's Health, Obstetric and Neonatal Nurses's Respectful Maternity Care Initiative

AWHONN's RMC initiative is an approach also designed to address to the relatively high and rising rates of maternal M&M, and significant inequities in maternal and infant outcomes for minoritized populations in the US.[22] As health care provider biases, explicit and implicit, and inconsistent provision of evidence-based care are known to be associated with adverse outcomes, the initiative's materials promote equitable access to evidence-based care while recognizing a patient's unique needs and preferences in order to consistently provide RMC for every patient, every time. The initiative includes a RMC Framework, Evidence-Based Clinical Practice Guideline, and an RMC Implementation Toolkit available on the AWHONN's website.[22] While AWHONN is a nursing organization, the practices and guidelines included in the RMC initiative are to be utilized by all-care team members within a birthing unit and implementation requires multi-disciplinary engagement and support that OB Hospitalists can provide.

Trauma-Informed Care

Trauma-informed care (TIC) is a patient-centered approach that recognizes in order to provide effective patient-care; it is necessary to understand a patient's background and life experiences. TIC has evolved greatly over the last half century, with an initial focus on post-traumatic stress disorder (PTSD) in war veterans in the 1960s to 70s to more broadly encompassing patients of all demographics in all health care realms.[23,24] Established by the Congress in the 1990s, The Substance Abuse and Mental Health Services Administration has since created a dynamic framework for defining trauma. This framework recognizes trauma results from "an event, series of events, or set of circumstances that is experienced by an individual as physically or emotionally harmful or life threatening and that has lasting adverse effects on the individual's functioning and mental, physical, social, emotional, or spiritual well-being."[23] The trauma-informed approach focuses on 5 core principles: safety, trustworthiness, choice, collaboration, and empowerment (**Fig. 2**).[23]

It is well-established that trauma traverses all demographics; however, distinct populations are at increased risk and experience higher rates of trauma in the US.[23] A National Comorbidity study in 2012 estimated that half of individuals identifying as women in the US will be exposed to a traumatic event in their lifetime.[25] Although studies found men have a greater risk of trauma, women are more likely to experience PTSD.[26] Women are also more likely than men to experience intimate partner violence (IPV), with recent data from the Centers for Disease Control and Prevention (CDC) reporting 1 in 3 women have experienced physical violence from a partner and 1 in 5 has experienced sexual violence.[27] Pregnant individuals are disproportionately affected by IPV with the highest prevalence of emotional abuse (30%), physical (15%), and sexual abuse (8%).[28] Research has further shown that IPV in gravidas is largely influenced by demographics, with non-Hispanic American Indian/Alaska Native, and black populations reporting increased prevalence of IPV during pregnancy.[29]

Given the personally sensitive nature of prenatal and intrapartum care, individuals may experience new or acute trauma, exacerbations of prior trauma, or realize unaddressed trauma. In their 2021 bulletin, the American College of Obstetrics and Gynecology (ACOG) recommends all obstetrician-gynecologists "implement universal screening for current trauma and a history of trauma."[30] ACOG further advises all health care providers to "screen for IPV at the initial prenatal visit, at least once per trimester, and during the postpartum visit."[31] These screening tools are designed to identify patients who may benefit from multidisciplinary resources during their perinatal period and enable a smooth transition from outpatient prenatal care to inpatient care on the L&D unit.

OB/GYN hospitalists play a fundamental role in setting the standard for establishing a trauma-informed environment and delivering trauma-sensitive care throughout the individual's inpatient stay (see **Fig. 2**). A trauma-sensitive approach for all pregnant patients empowers all the L&D team members (nurses, midwives, medical assistants, physicians, students, and other team members) to contribute to patient-centered care and improve safety, patient experience, and health outcomes.[31,32] Multiple guidelines

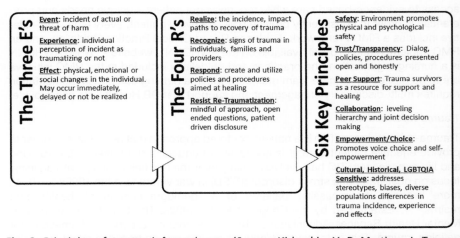

Fig. 2. Principles of trauma-informed care. (*Source:* Kislovskiy, Y, DeMartino, J, Trauma Informed Care for the OB/GYN Hospitalist, Journal of OB/GYN Hospital Medicine, Volume 2, Issue 3 (used with Permission).)

and examples exist for supporting TIC in OB/GYN, including team-based training, simulations, the development of universal screening questions in the electronic health record, hospital-led programs or initiatives, and utilizing community input and resources (**Fig. 3**). One specific program focused on TIC in the perinatal period is the M-Power program at Cleveland Clinic.

M-Power

M-Power is a program that provides perinatal care for pregnant individuals with a history of trauma.[33] The program was created at Cleveland Clinic by Patricia Gilbert, BSN, RN and Dusty Burke, MSN, RN, C-EFM and inspired by the book *When Survivors Give Birth* by Penny Simkin and Phyllis Klaus.[34] M-Power is entirely nursing-led and based on referrals. Health care providers can refer patients to the program at any stage of their pregnancy or patients can self-refer by directly calling the program or by responding to an automatic screening message sent via the electronic health record to every patient at 20 weeks gestational age.

After referrals are placed, M-Power nurses trained in TIC contact patients in the third trimester to discuss the L&D process in depth (including hospital tours) and create each patient's individualized birth plan. The plans are compiled in an "M-Power Consult" note that can be accessed by any provider who will be caring for the patient in the perinatal period. These consults detail individuals' needs during the birthing process, for example, what language to use or not to use while the patient is in labor, examples of potential triggers for patients, and other patient-specific information. Following delivery, M-Power coordinators connect patients with additional resources they may need in the postpartum period. At every milestone in perinatal care (pregnancy, birth, and postpartum), M-power supports and empowers birthing individuals to be directly involved in their plan of care, providing a safe space for their voices to be heard.

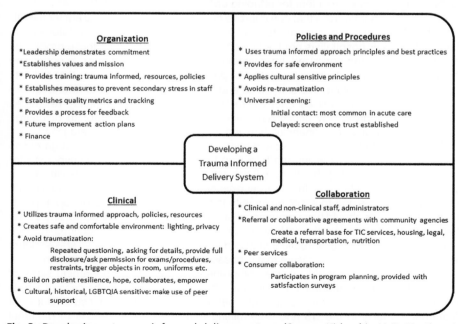

Fig. 3. Developing a trauma-informed delivery system. (*Source:* Kislovskiy, Y, DeMartino, J, Trauma Informed Care for the OB/GYN Hospitalist, Journal of OB/GYN Hospital Medicine, Volume 2, Issue 3 (used with Permission).)

EQUITY CONSIDERATIONS IN QUALITY & SAFETY
Optimizing Transitions of Care Between In-Patient Settings

Effective communication between care team members is essential at all times in OB. This is especially true during key transitions in care including transfer from triage or OB emergency department or antepartum to labor and delivery and with admission of patients from labor and delivery to postpartum. Strategies that can be utilized to optimize team communication during transitions of care include requiring standardized approaches to team huddles or safety "time-outs" during key transitions, which have been shown to be successful in improving perceptions of team communication and safety.[35] Units can specify transitions for which huddles must occur (admission, transfer to postpartum), team member involvement, and pertinent information that should be included at huddles (**Box 1**).[35]

Enhanced Discharge Planning

A significant proportion of maternal M&M and inequities in maternal outcomes occur in the postpartum period, therefore, there has been much attention on improving care in the "fourth trimester" in order to improve maternal outcomes.[36,37] Transitions to outpatient care in the postpartum period are vital in ensuring optimal health outcomes. ACOG has advised that "All women should ideally have contact with a maternal care provider within the first 3 weeks postpartum. This initial assessment should be followed-up with ongoing care as needed, concluding with a comprehensive postpartum visit no later than 12 weeks after birth."[37] ACOG also advises that patients with "chronic medical conditions, such as hypertensive disorders, obesity, diabetes, thyroid disorders, renal disease, mood disorders, and substance use disorders, should be counseled regarding the importance of timely follow-up with their OB/GYN or primary care providers for ongoing coordination of care."[36,37]

Many of the interventions that can improve care and outcomes are salient for the OB hospitalist as they can occur prior to discharge from a delivery or readmission hospitalization and OB hospitalists are the key advocates in assuring that these processes are implemented and optimized. Interventions that have shown promise in optimizing postpartum care include implementation of patient navigators to ensure that patients have necessary appointments scheduled and the resources needed to attend follow-up appointments, as well as referrals to "wrap around" or community resources necessary to address key social determinants of health needs prior to discharge from a hospitalization (eg, financial, housing, transportation, nutrition, etc.).[36,38]

Collaboration between OB-GYNs and primary care providers has been recognized as a key strategy in strengthening the transition between obstetric and primary care for women for and managing chronic conditions across the life course.[37] The in-patient hospitalization offers a vital opportunity to place necessary referrals to assure assistance with essential resources and to assist patients to facilitate scheduling of follow-up appointments. All patients should have required follow-up appointments scheduled, and all patients needing navigation should have appropriate referrals and connections in place prior to discharge from an in-patient stay and OB hospitalists can be vital stakeholders within a unit's leadership to assure that processes are in place for this to happen.

Lastly, all patients should receive comprehensive education on warning signs of complications and instructions on how and when to obtain care in the case of a suspected complication in the postpartum period. After a comprehensive review of maternal mortality in the US and determining that approximately 80% of maternal deaths are preventable, the CDC launched the "Hear Her" campaign 2022.[39] The campaign centers on raising "awareness of urgent maternal warning signs during

---

Box 1
Admission Huddle Components

- Name
- Age
- Gravidity and parity
- Gestational age of fetus
- Allergies
- Reason for admission
- Past medical history
- Past obstetric/gynecologic history
- Social history including alcohol, tobacco
- Illegal drug use
- Domestic violence
- Sexually transmitted diseases
- Laboratory results (blood type, group b streptococcus status, or other significant labs)
- Membrane status
- Most recent sterile vaginal examination
- Desire for intrauterine device or bilateral tubal ligation
- Fetal presentation on ultrasound
- Other concerns such as abnormal vital signs, fetal heart rate tracing, or pain
- Any barriers that may delay the woman's plan of care

---

and after pregnancy and improve communication between patients and their health care providers," and provides resources for patients, support persons, and health care providers to improve recognition and treatment of perinatal complications.[39] OB hospitalists should be engaged in ensuring that all patients are consistently receiving the information they need prior to discharge to appropriately identify complications and seek care when needed.

Peer Review or Adverse Event Debriefs

Direct medical care has been found to account for only 20% of variation in health outcomes, while the remaining 80% can be attributed to social determinants of health including income, education, nutrition, housing, basic amenities, discrimination, and access to health care.[19] Social determinants of health are especially important when considering inequities in health care outcomes for minoritized populations.[40] Common quality and safety processes at most facilities include peer review and adverse event debriefs. Both processes offer opportunities to improve on traditional approaches of primarily identifying issues with medical care as contributing to adverse events with expansion to also considering systemic and equity-related contributors. Inclusion of systemic and equity-related factors into quality and safety processes are essential in identifying and addressing underlying etiologies of adverse health outcomes, and OB hospitalists are again, as integral unit quality and safety leaders, ideally positioned as advocates for this process evolution.

In order to mitigate bias in the review process, a standardized and systematic approach should be taken to assess for factors that may have contributed to an outcome including system factors, medical care, provider-related factors, and equity-related factors. A sample standardized list of potential equity-related factors for inclusion is mentioned as follows (**Fig. 4**) and sample debrief (Appendix 1) and peer review (Appendix 2) forms that incorporate equity are included in appendices. A system should be implemented to ensure that all factors identified to be contributing to an adverse event are systematically tracked and addressed.

Of note, in an immediate review of an adverse event, the patient and support persons should be included. The event should be reviewed with them to promote communication, transparency, education, and collaboration, and their feedback on contributing factors and opportunities for improvement should be recorded and analyzed for process improvement.

Morbidity & Mortality Conferences

As with peer review and adverse event debrief processes, M&M conferences are a common quality and safety practice in most health care institutions. Traditional M&M conferences have focused analysis of individual provider practices, for example, surgical techniques or deviation from institutional care protocols that lead to an adverse outcome. M&M conferences can be another forum where OB/GYN hospitalists can advocate for inclusion, examination, discussion, and education surrounding equity-related and larger systemic factors that commonly contribute to adverse health outcomes, disparities in health outcomes, and for opportunities for systems improvement. Numerous health care systems around the US have incorporated equity-focused M&M conferences into their OB/GYN division's longitudinal quality and safety activities that can provide a template for divisions seeking to initiate the process. A sample structure for equity-focused M&M rounds is available in Appendix 3.[41]

Becoming Champions for Education in Diversity, Equity, and Inclusion

OB/GYN hospitalists are increasingly becoming leaders in education. This evolution has resulted from their consistent presence on L&D as they lead the orchestration of inpatient care. OB/GYN hospitalists are in a unique position to not only teach evidence-based practices, but to also be models and educators of diversity, equity, and inclusion (DEI) in patient-care. Key components to DEI education and simulation training include: self-reflection with bias training for educators and learners, building a diversified education and simulation team, creating safe spaces for learning, providing respectfully supported debriefing opportunities and community engagement in the creation of DEI education.[42–45]

- Access to healthcare: Transportation, financial, insurance, geographic barriers, difficulties with system navigation (making appointments, etc)
- Communication/Language: Communication difficulties due to language barriers, use of interpreters, deaf services/sign language interpreter
- Culture: Cultural practices/beliefs affecting preferences/care (provider preference, acceptance of blood products, preferences regarding medical interventions, etc)
- Social: Housing/Homelessness, past trauma, Intimate partner violence/abuse, mental health concerns, opioid/substance use disorders, social support
- Bias/Discrimination: Race/ethnicity, gender, age, weight, gender identity, sexual orientation, education, socioeconomic status, religion, disabilities

---

* These are examples of equity-related issues that may contribute to adverse events, but issues are not limited to those listed here.

Fig. 4. Equity considerations.

STRATEGIES FOR OBSTETRICS AND GYNECOLOGY HOSPITALISTS AS DIVERSITY, EQUITY, AND INCLUSION EDUCATORS TO NORMALIZE CONVERSATIONS REGARDING BIAS- AND EQUITY-RELATED CONSIDERATIONS: ADDRESSING BIAS

Implicit and explicit bias have been found to be highly prevalent in medical practitioners, to contribute to adverse experiences with health care and poor health outcomes, and to exacerbate inequities in health outcomes.[46,47] While conversations regarding bias and other equity-related concerns can be difficult, it is imperative that leaders in quality and safety in obstetric care environments such as OB/GYN hospitalists, be courageous and empowered to examine their own biases, address and normalize conversations around implicit bias and equity-related concerns to improve patient-care and outcomes.

Recommended approaches in addressing and discussing bias- and equity-related concerns include:

- Examining personal biases: Consistently question how personal biases may be affecting your actions.[48–50]
- Call out equity-related concerns when you see them: While this may be uncomfortable, ignoring bias or other equity-related concerns leads to perpetuation of the problem.[48]
- Remain calm, model the behavior you would like to see: Be sure that your delivery does not undermine the message you are trying to impart.[48]
- Create a safe space for discussion tough topics: Acknowledge that unconscious bias is a universal human condition rather than a personal flaw.[49]
- Assume best intentions: Reflect on intent versus impact of statements.[50]
- Be curious: Focus on questions to seek understanding and clarity rather than defending or convincing.[50]
- Be engaged and create the opportunity for discussion: Utilize active listening skills, practice empathy, and avoid "binary" mindsets (ie, right or wrong, good or bad).[49]
- Be comfortable with being uncomfortable: Learning requires growth, which can be painful, focus on encouragement rather than reassurance and accept an absence of closure.[49]
- Make clear when content or statements are unacceptable: Be aware of institutional policies and established procedures related to equity and inclusion.[51]
- Provide resources and education: Embrace the concept that "It's not about you" and leverage personal stories to promote consideration from the perspectives of others to help identify and eliminate personal biases.[50]
- Support anyone who is advocating: Give no outlet or connection for bias, instead encourage and promote camaraderie around inclusion.[49]
- Expect to make mistakes: Remember that everyone is learning, mistakes will happen and offer opportunities to learn and do better next time.[49]

STRATEGIES FOR OBSTETRICS AND GYNECOLOGY HOSPITALISTS AS DIVERSITY, EQUITY, AND INCLUSION EDUCATORS: DIVERSIFYING EDUCATORS, CREATING SAFE SPACES FOR LEARNING AND CREATING RELEVANCE THROUGH COMMUNITY

Diverse educational opportunities in DEI training exist and can encompass a variety of formats including interactive modules, didactic lectures, simulations, or a combination of these methods. Diversity in both educational opportunities and educators is the key to create an inclusive environment. Educators from varying backgrounds bring a rich tapestry of lived and professional experience to the educational process. It aids in creating safe spaces in which a variety of learners feel represented and supported throughout their educational experience. Educators are provided the opportunity to model behaviors and to provide diverse perspectives to support and answer learner questions.[44] Lastly, debriefing is a crucial component of the educational experience as it provides learners with a safe space to express themselves and to share insights with their peers and educators.[45,52] It also provides educators with the opportunity to share their own experiences and perspectives to attain a deeper understanding of their own biases and how those biases might impact their teaching practices. By creating open opportunities for discussion, educators can learn and grow, ultimately improving their effectiveness in ensuring that all learners feel heard, valued, and supported.[45,52,53] Lastly, incorporating community input in the development of DEI curriculum ensures that education is relevant to the daily practices of the OB/GYN hospitalist and supporting team. By involving community stakeholders, such as patients, families and community organizations, educators can tailor the curriculum to address the specific needs and challenges encountered in these health care settings. Moreover, involving the community promotes buy-in and encourages behavior modifications among health care professionals, ultimately improving patient-care and satisfaction.[43]

COMMUNITY INVOLVEMENT IN ELIMINATING INEQUITIES IN HEALTH OUTCOMES

Engaging patients and communities in quality improvement, governance, and interventions within health care systems, especially work centered on eliminating inequities in health outcomes, is vital in ensuring that interventions are meaningful, effective, and culturally appropriate.[54] Patients and community members can be engaged in selection, design, implementation, and evaluation of interventions, training, and programming through institutional community accountability panels that include a diverse representation of patients and community members and collaboration with community-based organizations working in the maternal and child health space. Patients and community members provide expertise on lived experience and community knowledge essential for health care systems in implementation of the most effective interventions and in quality assurance. Bi-directional sharing of information, expertise, and resources between health care institutions, patients, and community-based organizations promotes transparency, trust, collaboration, resource sharing, capacity building, broadening communication efforts, and community investment.[54]

OB hospitalists can advocate for engagement of patients and community members in the work and quality and safety processes of health care systems by assisting with formation of community accountability panels, by participating in local, state, and national DEI committees and perinatal health working groups, and by participating in and promoting local and institution community-based interventions and activities. The March of Dimes is a leading community-based organization that offers guidance on engagement of families and community members with health care organizations, as well as numerous opportunities for health care system, provider, and community member engagement and collaboration including multiple opportunities to participate in Mother Baby Action Network[55] working groups and local community-based activities such as annual fundraising activities, meet the midwives, and community baby showers.

SUMMARY

With roles as designated leaders on L&D and postpartum units, and as coordinators of multidisciplinary care teams, OB/GYN hospitalists are uniquely poised to act as advocates for initiatives to improve care delivery for obstetric patients. This review serves as a reference for evidence-based and innovative best practice strategies that OB/

GYN hospitalists may engage in, facilitate, and promote in reduction of severe maternal M&M, addressing leading contributors to maternal mortality, and eliminating disparities in obstetric and neonatal outcomes.

CLINICS CARE POINTS

- Following standardized evidence-baded practices has proven to be an effective strategy to decrease maternal morbidity and mortality.

- Meeting patients where they are, providing education, access to resources and partnering in their health care decision making process is an impactful strategy to reduce preventable causes of maternal mortality and near misses.

- To decrease preventable mortality during the postpartum period, it's essential to provide comprehensive discharge planning that addresses barriers to care, optimizes resources, and educates patients about early warning signs and when to seek care.

- Peer review, adverse event debriefing, and debriefing with the patient and their support system provide opportuniites to detect preventable causes of harm and reinforce a culture of safe, equitable and inclusive care.

DISCLOSURE

The authors of this publication, J. DeMartino, M.Y. Katsuki and M.R. Ansbro have no financial or commercial conflicts of interest or funding sources to disclose.

REFERENCES

1. Hoyert D. Maternal mortality rates in the United States, 2021. National Center for Health Statistics (U.S.); 2023. https://doi.org/10.15620/cdc:124678.
2. United States Government Accountability Office (GAO), Report to Congressional Addressees. Maternal Health: Outcomes Worsened and Disparities Persisted During the Pandemic. Published online October 2022.
3. Fleszar LG, Bryant AS, Johnson CO, et al. Trends in State-Level Maternal Mortality by Racial and Ethnic Group in the United States. JAMA 2023;330(1):52–61.
4. Fink DA, Kilday D, Cao Z, et al. Trends in Maternal Mortality and Severe Maternal Morbidity During Delivery-Related Hospitalizations in the United States, 2008 to 2021. JAMA Netw Open 2023;6(6):e2317641.
5. Fischer F, Lange K, Klose K, et al. Barriers and Strategies in Guideline Implementation-A Scoping Review. Healthc Basel Switz 2016;4(3):36.
6. Shields LE, Wiesner S, Klein C, et al. Use of Maternal Early Warning Trigger tool reduces maternal morbidity. Am J Obstet Gynecol 2016;214(4):527.e1–6.
7. Mhyre JM, D'Oria R, Hameed AB, et al. The maternal early warning criteria: a proposal from the national partnership for maternal safety. Obstet Gynecol 2014; 124(4):782–6.
8. Alliance For Innovation On Maternal Health. AIM Patient Safety Bundles. eModule 1 Maternal Early Warning System (MEWS). Available at: https://saferbirth.org/.
9. ACOG Committee Opinon No. 766: Approaches to Limit Intervention During Labor and Birth. Available at: https://www.acog.org/clinical/clinical-guidance/committee-opinion/articles/2019/02/approaches-to-limit-intervention-during-labor-and-birth. [Accessed 1 February 2024].
10. Stephenson J. Rate of First-time Cesarean Deliveries on the Rise in the US. JAMA Health Forum 2022;3(7):e222824.

11. Total cesarean deliveries by maternal race/ethnicity: United States, 2019-2021 Average. March of Dimes | PeriStats. Available at: https://www.marchofdimes. org/peristats/data?reg=99&top=8&stop=356&lev=1&slev=1&obj=1. [Accessed 1 February 2024].

12. Carlson NS, Carlson MS, Erickson EN, et al. Disparities by race/ethnicity in unplanned cesarean birth among healthy nulliparas: a secondary analysis of the nuMoM2b dataset. BMC Pregnancy Childbirth 2023;23(1):342.

13. ACOG Committee Opinion No. 716: Cesarean Delivery on Maternal Request. 2019. Available at: https://www.acog.org/clinical/clinical-guidance/committee-opinion/articles/2019/01/cesarean-delivery-on-maternal-request. [Accessed 1 February 2024].

14. California Maternal Quality Care Collaborative (CMQCC). Toolkit to Support Vaginal Birth and Reduce Primary Cesareans | California Maternal Quality Care Collaborative. Available at: https://www.cmqcc.org/VBirthToolkitResource. [Accessed 1 February 2024].

15. ACOG. ACOG Practice Bulletin No. 231: Multifetal Gestations Twin Triplet and Higher-Order Multifetal Pregnancies. 2021. Available at: https://www.acog.org/clinical/clinical-guidance/practice-bulletin/articles/2021/06/multifetal-gestations-twin-triplet-and-higher-order-multifetal-pregnancies. [Accessed 1 February 2024].

16. ACOG. ACOG Clinical Practice Guideline No. 8: First and Second Stage Labor Management. 2024. Available at: https://www.acog.org/clinical/clinical-guidance/clinical-practice-guideline/articles/2024/01/first-and-second-stage-labor-management. [Accessed 1 February 2024].

17. ACOG. ACOG Practice Advisory: Counseling Regarding Approach to Delivery After Cesarean and the Use of a Vaginal Birth After Cesarean Calculator. Available at: https://www.acog.org/clinical/clinical-guidance/practice-advisory/articles/2021/12/counseling-regarding-approach-to-delivery-after-cesarean-and-the-use-of-a-vaginal-birth-after-cesarean-calculator. [Accessed 1 February 2024].

18. CDC. Mistreatment during maternity care. Centers for Disease Control and Prevention; 2023. Available at: https://www.cdc.gov/vitalsigns/respectful-maternity-care/index.html. [Accessed 31 January 2024].

19. Hood CM, Gennuso KP, Swain GR, et al. County Health Rankings: Relationships Between Determinant Factors and Health Outcomes. Am J Prev Med 2016;50(2): 129–35.

20. Hüner B, Derksen C, Schmiedhofer M, et al. Reducing preventable adverse events in obstetrics by improving interprofessional communication skills – Results of an intervention study. BMC Pregnancy Childbirth 2023;23(1):55.

21. Ariadne Labs. Delivery decisions intitiative. Ariadne Labs. Available at: https://www.ariadnelabs.org/delivery-decisions-initiative/. [Accessed 31 January 2024].

22. Association of Women's Health, Obstetric and Neonatal Nursesadmin. Respectful maternity care implementation toolkit. AWHONN. Available at: https://www.awhonn.org/respectful-maternity-care-implementation-toolkit/. [Accessed 29 January 2024].

23. Subtance Abuse and Mental Health ServicesAdministration. SAMHSA's Concept of Trauma and Guidance for a Trauma-InformedApproach. HHS Publication No. (SMA) 14-4884. Rockville, MD: Substance Abuse and Mental Health Services Administration, 2014.

24. Harris M and Fallot R, Editors. Using Trauma Theory to Design Service Systems. New Directions for Mental Health Services 2011; San Francisco: Jossey-Bass.

25. Mitchell KS, Mazzeo SE, Schlesinger MR, et al. Comorbidity of partial and sub-threshold ptsd among men and women with eating disorders in the national co-morbidity survey-replication study. Int J Eat Disord 2012;45(3):307–15.

26. Olff M. Sex and gender differences in post-traumatic stress disorder: an update. Eur J Psychotraumatol 2017;8(sup4):1351204.

27. CDC. Fast Facts: Preventing Intimate Partner Violence. 2023. Available at: https://www.cdc.gov/violenceprevention/intimatepartnerviolence/fastfact.html.   [Accessed 31 January 2024].

28. Huecker MR, King KC, Jordan GA, et al. Domestic Violence. In: StatPearls. StatPearls Publishing; 2024. Available at: http://www.ncbi.nlm.nih.gov/books/NBK499891/. [Accessed 31 January 2024].

29. Chisholm CA, Bullock L, Ferguson JEJ. Intimate partner violence and pregnancy: epidemiology and impact. Am J Obstet Gynecol 2017;217(2):141–4.

30. Caring for Patients Who Have Experienced Trauma: ACOG Committee Opinion Summary. Number 825. Obstet Gynecol 2021;137(4):757–8.

31. ACOG Committee Opinion No. 518: Intimate partner violence. Obstet Gynecol 2012;119(2 Pt 1):412–7.

32. Nagle-Yang S, Sachdeva J, Zhao LX, et al. Trauma-Informed Care for Obstetric and Gynecologic Settings. Matern Child Health J 2022;26(12):2362–9.

33. Cleveland Clinic's Specialized Perinatal Service for Survivors – Consult QD. Available at: https://consultqd.clevelandclinic.org/cleveland-clinics-specialized-peri-natal-service-for-survivors/. [Accessed 31 January 2024].

34. Simkin Penny, Klaus Phyllis. When Survivors give birth. 1st edition. Classic Day Publishing; 2004.

35. O'Rourke K, Teel J, Nicholls E, et al. Improving Staff Communication and Transitions of Care Between Obstetric Triage and Labor and Delivery. J Obstet Gynecol Neonatal Nurs 2018;47(2):264–72.

36. Phillips SEK, Celi AC, Wehbe A, et al. Mobilizing the fourth trimester to improve population health: interventions for postpartum transitions of care. Am J Obstet Gynecol 2023;229(1):33–8.

37. ACOG Committee Opinon No. 736: Optimizing postpartum care. Obstet Gynecol 2018;131(5):e140–50.

38. Essien UR, Molina RL, Lasser KE. Strengthening the postpartum transition of care to address racial disparities in maternal health. J Natl Med Assoc 2019;111(4): 349–51.

39. CDC. CDC's hear her campaign. Centers for Disease Control and Prevention; 2022. Available at: https://www.cdc.gov/hearher/index.html. [Accessed 31 January 2024].

40. Fan LL, Sheth SS, Pettker CM. Pilot Implementation of a Health Equity Checklist to Improve the Identification of Equity-Related Adverse Events. Obstet Gynecol 2022;140(4):667–73.

41. Reisinger-Kindle K, Dethier D, Wang V, et al. Health Equity Morbidity and Mortality Conferences in Obstetrics and Gynecology. Obstet Gynecol 2021;138(6): 918–23.

42. Walshe N, Condon C, Gonzales RA, et al. Cultural Simulations, Authenticity, Focus, and Outcomes: A Systematic Review of the Healthcare Literature. Clin Simul Nurs 2022;71:65–81.

43. Tjia J, Pugnaire M, Calista J, et al. Using Simulation-Based Learning with Standardized Patients (SP) in an Implicit Bias Mitigation Clinician Training Program. J Med Educ Curric Dev 2023;10:23821205231175033.

44. Vora S, Dahlen B, Adler M, et al. Recommendations and Guidelines for the Use of Simulation to Address Structural Racism and Implicit Bias. Simul Healthc J Soc Simul Healthc 2021;16(4):275–84.

45. Miller JL, Bryant K, Park C. Moving From "Safe" to "Brave" Conversations: Committing to Antiracism in Simulation. Simul Healthc J Soc Simul Healthc 2021;16(4):231–2.

46. Marcelin JR, Siraj DS, Victor R, et al. The Impact of Unconscious Bias in Health-care: How to Recognize and Mitigate It. J Infect Dis 2019;220(220 Suppl 2): S62–73.

47. Vela MB, Erondu AI, Smith NA, et al. Eliminating Explicit and Implicit Biases in Health Care: Evidence and Research Needs. Annu Rev Public Health 2022;43: 477–501.

48. Williams AL. How to speak up if you see bias at work. Harv Bus Rev. Available at: https://hbr.org/2017/01/how-to-speak-up-if-you-see-bias-at-work. [Accessed 1 May 2017].

49. A Leader's guide to talking about bias. Harvard Graduate School of Education. Available at: https://www.gse.harvard.edu/ideas/usable-knowledge/20/08/ leaders-guide-talking-about-bias. [Accessed 3 August 2020].

50. Panel E. 14 Ways Leaders can Effectively address unconscious biases in others. Forbes. Available at: https://www.forbes.com/sites/forbescoachescouncil/2021/ 10/20/14-ways-leaders-can-effectively-address-unconscious-biases-in-others/? sh=37ad41fa4b08. [Accessed 20 October 2021].

51. UNC School of Medicine Office of Diversity, Equity, and Inclusion. Implicit bias | Office of Diversity, Equity, and Inclusion. Office of Diversity, Equity, and Inclusion. Available at: https://www.med.unc.edu/inclusion/justice-equity-diversity-and-in-clusion-j-e-d-i-toolkit/implicit-bias/. [Accessed 25 May 2023].

52. Eppich W, Cheng A. Promoting Excellence and Reflective Learning in Simulation (PEARLS): development and rationale for a blended approach to health care simulation debriefing. Simul Healthc J Soc Simul Healthc 2015;10(2):106–15.

53. Broaching Race and Racism in Debriefing and Team Simulations (Part 1). Center for Medical Simulation. Available at: https://harvardmedsim.org/resources/ weekly-webinars-aug-05-2020-broaching-race-and-racism-in-debriefing-and-team-simulations-part-1/. [Accessed 1 February 2024].

54. Meadows AR, Byfield R, Bingham D, et al. Strategies to Promote Maternal Health Equity: The Role of Perinatal Quality Collaboratives. Obstet Gynecol 2023; 142(4):821.

55. March of Dimes. March of Dimes: Mom and Baby Action Network. Available at: https://ignitingimpacttogether.marchofdimes.org/mom-and-baby-action-network. [Accessed 1 February 2024].

APPENDIX 1: OBSTETRIC TEAM DEBRIEFING FORM

Patient Label

Debriefing is a process addressing human factors and system issues to improve the team's response for the next event. Debriefing is a non-judgmental learning experience for the team.

Date of Event: _____   Time of Event: _____   Time of Debrief: _____

Location of Event: _____

Type of Event:

□ HTN (Sustained severe hypertension unresponsive to treatment with maximum doses of acute antihypertensive agents)
□ Obstetric Hemorrhage >4 units RBC transfused and/or transfer to ICU
□ Maternal Transfer to ICU   □ Shoulder Dystocia
□ Maternal Death   □ Uterine Rupture
□ Maternal Sepsis   □ Emergent/STAT/Crash C-Section
□ Other: _____

Members of the Team Present for Debrief:

□ Team Lead/ Primary MD _____   □ RN_____
□ Anesthesia Personnel _____   □ RN_____
□ Maternal Fetal Medicine_____   □ CNM_____
□ Neonatology Personnel _____   □ NM/Charge Nurse_____
□ Resident_____   □ PCNA _____
□ OB/Surgical Tech_____   □ Other _____

When completed please turn this form into _____

Review of how the obstetric emergency was managed:

Identify what went well: (Check if yes)	Identify Opportunities for improvement: "Human Factors" (Check if yes)	Identify opportunities for improvement: "System issues" (Check if yes)	Did any Equity- Related factors/barriers contribute to the event? (Check if yes)
□ Communication	□ Communication	□ Equipment	□ Access to Healthcare
□ Role Clarity (leader/supporting roles identified and assigned)	□ Role Clarity (leader/supporting roles identified and assigned)	□ Medication	□ Communication/Language
□ Teamwork	□ Teamwork	□ Blood Product Availability	□ Culture
□ Situational Awareness	□ Situational Awareness	□ Inadequate support (in unit or other areas of the hospital)	□ Social
□ Decision- Making	□ Decision- Making	□ Delays in transporting the patient (within hospital or to another facility)	□ Bias/Discrimination
□ Communication with Patient/Family	□ Communication with Patient/Family	□ Other_____	□ Other_____
□ Other_____	□ Other_____		

For Identified Issues, Fill in Below (actions/person responsible are optional at time of debrief)

ISSUE	WHO IDENTIFIED ISSUE? (Choose all that apply)	ACTIONS TO BE TAKEN	PERSON ASSIGNED FOR FOLLOW UP
	___ Nurse ___ OB Provider ___ Anesthesia ___ NICU/Peds ___ Other		
	___ Nurse ___ OB Provider ___ Anesthesia ___ NICU/Peds ___ Other		
	___ Nurse ___ OB Provider ___ Anesthesia ___ NICU/Peds ___ Other		

APPENDIX 2: OB/GYN PEER REVIEW FORM

Situation:

Reason for Referral to Peer Review:

Background:

Pertinent Patient Descriptors (Age, Gravidity/Parity, Race/Ethnicity, Language, Gestational Age):

Pertinent Patient History (PMH, PSH, OB/Gyn Hx, Medications):

Hospital course/Timeline of events related to the event:

Pertinent labs and imaging:

Procedural details related to complication (if applicable):

Management of the event:

Involvement of other services (if applicable):

Details/Discussion with Provider(s) involved (if applicable):

Assessment:

Appropriate history taking, assessment, examinations?

Appropriate diagnostic workup?

Abnormal findings addressed appropriately?

Contributing Factors (please check all that apply):

Individual	Technical/Environmental	Diagnostic	Treatment
□ Knowledge □ Experience □ Evidence-based practice	□ Equipment □ Unit Environment □ Staffing □ Delays	□ Labs □ Imaging □ Procedures	□ Medication □ Procedures
Communication	Organizational/Systemic	Patient	Equity-Related
□ Documentation □ Care coordination/continuity □ Escalation □ Team communication □ Professionalism □ Communication with Patient/Support persons	□ Rules/Policies	□ Condition □ Comorbidities □ Distress	□ Access to Healthcare □ Communication/Language □ Culture □ Social □ Bias/Discrimination

Other Factors:_____

Please Provide Recommendations:

Classification:

Learning Points: How could the event have been prevented or management improved?:

Recommended Actions (Departmental improvements, System concerns, Provider concerns):

APPENDIX 3: PROPOSED OBSTETRICS AND GYNECOLOGY EQUITY MORBIDITY AND MORTALITY CONFERENCES

- Proposal for Conferences to be held [monthly, quarterly, bi-annually, etc.].
- Invitation to multidisciplinary team members to attend Conferences.
- Proposed cases for inclusion to be reviewed by [Quality & Safety Leadership, DEI Committee, etc.] to determine appropriateness and related literature and didactic components.
- Cases to be presented by [Resident Physicians, Medical Students, Staff Physicians, Quality & Safety Team, etc].
- Discussions to be facilitated by Staff trained in DEI discussion facilitation.

Goals/Objectives:

- Examine systematic inequities in health care
- Improve quality of care and patient experience
- Expand medical knowledge base
- Improve interpersonal communication skills and professionalism
- Generate system-level quality improvement initiatives
- Create a Just Culture

Cases For Inclusion (May include but not limited to):

- Economic Barriers
- Systemic Barriers
- Social Barriers
- Language Barriers
- Cultural Barriers
- Policy Barriers
- Community Barriers
- Inequities in Treatment or Diagnosis
- Inequities in Outcomes
- Inequities Related to Race/Ethnicity
- Inequities Related to Gender
- Inequities Related to Sexual Orientation/Gender Identity
- Unconscious Bias
- Discrimination
- Reproductive justice

Proposed Conference Framework (1-Hour Session):

- "Just Culture" Introduction
- Patient-Centered Case Presentation
- Relevant Literature Review
- Didactic Component
- Facilitated Discussion & Reflection
- Post-session debriefs, evaluation & feedback [Participant surveys, facilitator huddle, leadership update, etc.]

Gynecologic Hospitalists
Expanding the "G" in the Obstetrics and Gynecologic Hospitalist Role

Jennifer L. Eaton, DO*, Vicki R. Reed, MD,
Monique Yoder Katsuki, MD, MPH

KEYWORDS

- OB/GYN hospitalist • Gynecologic emergency • Quality and safety metrics
- Resident education

KEY POINTS

- The obstetrics and gynecology hospitalists' primary role is to care for obstetric and gynecologic patients in the emergency room and in the hospital.
- The focus for gynecologic hospitalist will be to achieve and support advanced skills in urgent and emergency gynecologic care, inpatient and intraoperative consultation, medical education, and monitoring quality and safety metrics.
- The hospitalist takes an educational role by providing guidance to and mentorship to peers, medical students, and residents.

INTRODUCTION

The obstetrics and gynecology (OB/GYN) hospitalist (OBGH) model was first proposed in 2003 and has been defined by the Society of OB/GYN Hospitalists as "an obstetrician/gynecologist who has focused their professional practice on care of the hospitalized woman."[1,2] Many benefits have been associated with OBGH providers including improved patient satisfaction, patient safety, and physician well-being/decreased fatigue.[3] The role of the OBGH stemmed from the need to improve patient safety on the labor and delivery unit and physician work-life balance.[3]

There is a broad range of roles the OBGH may have depending on the type of care model hospitals utilize, but the primary duties typically include caring for hospitalized patients, managing obstetric emergencies, and providing urgent gynecologic care and consultation in the emergency department (ED) and for non-OB/GYN hospital inpatient services.[1,2] Hospitalists coordinate management throughout the continuum of patient care in the hospital, often seeing a patient in the ED, monitoring them

Cleveland Clinic, Obstetrics and Gynecology Institute, A81, 9500 Euclid Avenue, Cleveland, OH 44195, USA
* Corresponding author.
E-mail address: eatonj2@ccf.org

Obstet Gynecol Clin N Am 51 (2024) 559–566
https://doi.org/10.1016/j.ogc.2024.05.004
0889-8545/24/© 2024 Elsevier Inc. All rights reserved, including those for text and data mining, AI training, and similar technologies.

obgyn.theclinics.com

throughout the full course of inpatient care including indicated surgical procedure(s), and coordinating post-acute follow-up.

The OBGH must have expertise in acute inpatient obstetric and gynecologic medicine and the positive effects of this expertise have been documented across different hospital systems as noted earlier.[1,2] While the spectrum of care of the OBGH includes both OB and GYN, most of the literature currently available focuses on care models and outcomes related to OB.[2,4,5] While most studies utilize the term hospitalist which includes hospitalists, nocturnists, and laborists, this document will refer to OBHs as hospitalists focusing on OB and GYNHs as hospitalists focusing on GYN. This article will highlight the role of the GYNH and their role in the OBGH model of care.[3]

GYNECOLOGIC HOSPITALIST ROLES AND RESPONSIBILITIES

The GYNH functions as part of the OBGH team, specifically caring for GYN patients in the traditional ED, hospital consultations, and urgent surgical add-on cases. In some institutes, the role of the GYNH will include care for obstetric patients less than 20 weeks' gestation and patients up to 6 weeks postpartum. GYNHs provide 24/7 coverage for gynecologic needs in the hospital which improves efficiency of triage, admissions, consultation, initiation and implementation of care plans, and discharge planning.[6] GYNHs may be providers who have an inpatient role only or who are part of a hybrid model where they provide care in the GYNH role part of their time and also have either an outpatient clinical role or an OBGH role. Having a dedicated provider in the GYNH role expedites action on testing and imaging results to improve patient care.[3] The GYNH is available to communicate and coordinate care with providers in other specialties and to plan care visits with patients and support persons. The GYNH will commonly care for patients with acute gynecologic diagnoses such as pelvic pain, abnormal uterine bleeding (AUB), vaginal discharge, vulvar and labial masses, ectopic pregnancy, ovarian torsion, ovarian cyst rupture, vulvar abscesses, missed/incomplete miscarriages, pregnancy of unknown location (PUL), sexually transmitted infections (STIs), pelvic inflammatory disease, and tubo-ovarian abscess. Common procedures the GYNH may perform include manual uterine evacuation at the bedside, dilation and curettage, and laparoscopy. Reduced time to treatment and surgical intervention, and operating room (OR) efficiency in gynecologic emergencies are key benefits of the GYNH as the surgeon is readily available onsite and is not juggling outpatient responsibilities. As part of the OBGH team, the GYNH may also utilize their OB knowledge and skills, for example, to assist during OB emergencies or with complex cesarean sections.

The day of the GYNH should begin with a direct physician-to-physician hand off from their colleague who completed the prior shift. This handoff is a verbal complement to a detailed written handoff tool in the electronic medical record and is essential in optimizing communication and effective coordination of care. The GYNH should also communicate with the OB team to understand the current state and needs of the obstetric unit. Rounding on inpatient GYN patients with modification to care plans as needed is another essential part of daily expectations, as well as communicating regarding care plans with the patient, support persons, consultative services, and nursing teams. The GYNH is often also responsible for new inpatient consultations, ED consultations and admissions, and acceptance of patient transfers to the hospital. The GYNH may also work with a team of physician assistants and/or advanced practice registered nurses, providing supervision of practice, back up, consultation regarding care plans, and intervention when escalation of care is needed. The GYNH is dedicated to hospital care and contributes to seamless transitions of care.

For example, when a GYNH evaluates patients who are pregnant and less than 20 weeks gestational age in ED or triage settings and patients require admission, the GYNH provides a comprehensive handoff to the maternal fetal medicine provider who will manage subsequent inpatient care. When patients are discharged from the hospital, ED or OB ED, outpatient follow-up is facilitated by the GYNH to assure efficient transitions of care and appropriate follow-up.

DEVELOPING A GYNECOLOGY HOSPITAL PROGRAM AND ASSOCIATED HOSPITAL RESOURCES

The development of the OBGH role improves access for patients seeking outpatient OB care, allowing outpatient OB/GYN providers more time in the office, and the GYN hospitalist role provides a similar benefit. The addition of advanced practice providers to outpatient care models also increases the volume of patients with potential emergent, inpatient GYN needs that the GYNH can help care for. Implementation of a GYNH model does require a practice with a patient volume to drive the need for a provider to be dedicated to this role.

In hospitals where the volume of gynecologic emergencies may not support a dedicated GYNH model, the presence of OBGHs becomes crucial. OBGHs are adept at managing both obstetric and gynecologic emergencies within the hospital setting. While their primary focus often is on obstetric care, they are trained to handle a wide range of gynecologic issues that may arise in the hospital, including emergencies.

In this context, OBGHs act as a bridge between outpatient OB/GYN providers and the hospital setting. When faced with gynecologic emergencies, they can step in to provide immediate care, stabilizing patients and initiating necessary treatments while coordinating with outpatient OB/GYN specialists for further management. This collaborative approach ensures seamless continuity of care, with the OBGH serving as the frontline responder in urgent situations.

The collaborative relationship between OBGHs and outpatient OB/GYN specialists is strengthened by the assurance of medical and surgical backup. Should complex cases arise, OB/GYN specialists are available to provide additional expertise and support, ensuring comprehensive care for patients across the continuum from outpatient to inpatient settings.

Medical facilities must provide comprehensive health services to support this model of care. The most important factor in developing a GYNH program is having leadership support and physician champions to ensure necessary services are in place to provide appropriate and timely care.[7,8] This includes ensuring diagnostic imaging capability with 24/7 availability of pelvic/transvaginal ultrasound and computed tomography scans, laboratory services including blood testing (complete blood counts, coagulation studies, chemistry panels, serum human chorionic gonadotropin levels, STI testing, and cultures), testing for vaginal and cervical infections, and pathology capabilities to evaluate uterine sampling. Availability of a blood bank is essential in ensuring access to blood products in case of hemorrhage. Coordination with the inpatient pharmacy is also vital to ensure availability of specific medications commonly required for GYN emergencies such as methotrexate, tranexamic acid, misoprostol, estrogen, and progesterone. The medical center must also have surgical capabilities with 24/7 anesthesia availability, appropriate equipment, and a skilled surgical OR team. Consultation services must be available for complex patient care such as intensive care unit teams, cardiology, pulmonology, urology, and infectious disease.

THE GYNECOLOGIC HOSPITALIST'S ROLE IN QUALITY IMPROVEMENT AND SAFETY

The GYNH is in a uniquely optimal role to allow for recognition of opportunities to improve quality of care, care delivery, and patient safety (**Fig. 1**). The GYNH plays a critical role in identifying quality improvement needs within a unit and care system, and guiding implementation of evidence-based best practices, and therefore must remain up to date with new guidelines and provide consistent evidence-based care. This includes development of gynecologic medicine by researching, developing, and implementing protocols and order sets for standardization of care. Standardization of medical care has been shown to lead to improved patient outcomes, and improved equity in outcomes for patients identifying with historically marginalized groups, and OBGHs can serve as a driving force behind the implementation of evidence-based care protocols and best practice recommendations.[9] For example, standardized care paths for management of headache or hyperemesis in the first trimester of pregnancy can be instituted to optimize initiation of patient care, with the goal of improved patient satisfaction and decreased length of stay. OBGHs can also collaborate with infectious disease and pharmacy teams to guide selection of appropriate antibiotic choices to avoid antibiotic resistance given local resistance profiles, and adjust recommendations when changes occur. Also, standard operating procedures for documenting packing for vulvar infection and drainage can avoid retained foreign bodies. The important role the OBGH can play in implementing newly available innovative devices and care practices has also been noted in the literature.[3]

As a central coordinator of inpatient care, it is essential that the GYNH develops optimal skills and practices in communication. Effective patient handoffs in transitions of care, updates on progress, and clear follow-up instructions between GYNH and patients, nurses, and other health care providers are vital to maintain patient safety.[5,7,9] Accountability and collaboration between providers in inpatient and outpatient settings is also vital in optimizing management for OB and GYN diagnoses with a potential for acute deterioration that require close surveillance and appropriate follow-up such as PUL and adnexal masses. For instance, patients with PUL must have short-interval, structured evaluation of laboratory and ultrasound findings to help prevent ruptured ectopic pregnancies. Appropriate and timely outpatient follow-up can be coordinated, and necessary patient education can be provided by the GYNH for these patients to assure optimal care and avoidance of adverse outcomes.

Staying informed about current quality-reporting metrics and the status of facility-specific patient outcomes is essential for the GYNH to meet established standards.

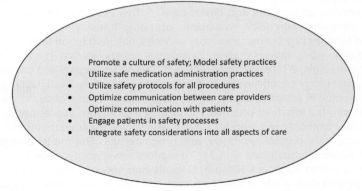

- Promote a culture of safety; Model safety practices
- Utilize safe medication administration practices
- Utilize safety protocols for all procedures
- Optimize communication between care providers
- Optimize communication with patients
- Engage patients in safety processes
- Integrate safety considerations into all aspects of care

Fig. 1. Gynecologic hospitalists' considerations for patient safety.[10]

In addition to benefits for patient care, quality outcomes are becoming publicly reported, and reimbursement is tied to outcomes.[7] These factors drive process change and standardization of practice models and the GYNH can leverage these factors to lead quality improvement and safety initiatives.

Additionally, inequities in treatment and outcomes for gynecologic emergencies such as ectopic pregnancy are well documented.[11] Evidence demonstrates that "disparities in gynecologic emergency care have previously been described at the patient level. Lower rates of methotrexate administration for tubal ectopic pregnancies have been noted in populations of patients with Medicaid insurance or no insurance, as have lower rates of tube-conserving surgical approaches in Black patients and populations of patients with low incomes."[11] OBGHs should maintain an awareness of facility and system-specific patient outcomes, as well as disparities in outcomes for vulnerable populations, in order to facilitate targeted interventions designed to eliminate gaps in equity.

As noted in the Introduction, there is some evidence that OBGH models improve patient satisfaction and clinical outcomes such as cesarean section rates.[12,13] Limited research that is available has shown that GYNH models can improve time to evaluation, treatment, and subsequent outcomes for GYN emergencies.[6] As most of the available research regarding the impacts of OBGH models of care is centered on effects on OB outcomes, there is an urgent need for OBGHs to engage in and generate additional research to better understand the impact and implications of OBGH models related to patient outcomes, especially GYNH models. Acute gynecologic conditions are common; it is estimated that 20% to 30% of women will experience AUB at some point in their lifetime, and this is a common presentation in emergency care settings.[14] *Gynecologic emergencies can be life-threatening, cause loss of fertility, and result in severe morbidity.*[14] Despite this, there is a limited amount of data related to gynecologic emergencies available in the literature as well as very limited research related to optimization of care in gynecologic emergencies compared to obstetric emergencies. One study has proposed a framework for collection and analysis of data regarding GYN emergencies to promote quality improvement that GYNH may adapt for quality improvement in the systems they work within (**Fig. 2**).

SIMULATION

Simulation has been well established as the gold standard for team readiness for, and optimal performance in, emergency situations. Simulated learning environments can range from low fidelity to high fidelity with a wide range of simple or technically complex models, or standardized patients. Another effective model for simulation is clinical site team training.[16] While the OBH's role in simulation may focus on hypertensive emergencies or OB hemorrhage, the GYNH can take the lead in facilitating emergency simulations focused on gynecologic diagnoses. An excellent opportunity for the GYNH to improve team readiness is in coordinating and facilitating multidisciplinary simulations that focus on stabilizing patients with acute GYN diagnoses (ie, acute bleeding with miscarriage management, vascular injury during laparoscopy) in the ED to expedite surgical intervention. Team training simulation can assist in identifying potential points for error, building comradery and interdisciplinary collaborative relationships, and increasing confidence in teamwork (**Fig. 3**).

EDUCATION

Education is multifaceted for the GYNH. They must stay current with guidelines and participate in peer review and collaborative and/or physician advisor groups to continually keep system practice guidelines and care protocols up to date. Trainees' learning

1. Tracking Conditions
   a. Define gynecologic emergencies for surveillance (i.e., Ectopic Pregnancy, Emergent Abnormal Uterine Bleeding, Miscarriage with Complications, Ovarian Torsion)
   b. Define and track "near miss" gynecologic emergency cases (cases with severe morbidity)
   c. Track fatalities related to gynecologic emergencies
2. Case Review for Critical Factors
   a. Time to diagnosis
      i. Assess for delays in diagnosis
      ii. Assess for errors in diagnosis
   b. Time to treatment
      i. Assess for delays in diagnosis
   c. Adherence of diagnosis and treatment to evidence-based, system guidelines/protocols
3. Practice Improvement
   a. Develop data collection process
      i. Regular review of data
      ii. Identify opportunities for improvement
   b. Develop evidence-based, best practice guidelines/protocols
      i. Update regularly
      ii. Ensure dissemination and accessibility

Fig. 2. Framework for quality improvement for the management of gynecologic emergencies.[15]

has been linked to faculty expertise and the longitudinal learning required by the GYNH is modeled for residents, students, and advanced practice providers.[19] Utilization of educational modalities via online modules or in-person classes covering communication, high-quality care, equitable and just care, respect for colleagues, and understanding of clinical guidelines is important to standardize and optimize care for all patients. Hospitalists have been shown to be effective educators by learners and the GYNH can serve as the point person for educational activities for all learners in the hospital setting.[19] This can include coverage of a specific list of topics for residents on rotation; additionally, topics can be covered as clinical examples occur. In academic medical settings, the GYNH also works closely with residents to advance their surgical skills and provide constructive feedback on clinical and surgical care. And the GYNH serves as an educator and consultant for colleagues who may need additional expertise in the OR. Provision of collegial support and guidance,

- Optimize transitions of care from out of hospital to inpatient, between units
- Ensure ready availability of appropriate emergency supplies (i.e., crash carts)
- Development of "rapid response" team and protocols
- Implement utilization of early warning systems (i.e., MEWS)
- Utilize standard communication tools for emergencies (i.e., SBAR)
- Consistently conduct post-event debriefs
- Implement longitudinal multidisciplinary emergency simulation education
- Participate in system safety processes (i.e., peer review, quality improvement collaboratives)

Fig. 3. Key tools for the gynecologic hospitalists in emergency preparedness.[17,18]

and mentorship for medical students, residents, and peers is another way the GYNH can serve in an educational capacity.[20]

SUMMARY

The GYNH is integral to the OBGH team, specializing in caring for GYN patients across various hospital settings. They care for a range of gynecologic diagnoses and are skilled with procedures such as dilation and curettage, and laparoscopy. They are integral to incorporating effective and comprehensive communication into patient rounds, consultations, and transitions of care to ensure optimal outcomes. Collaborating across specialties, GYNHs serve in a key coordinating role to ensure effective patient management, implementation of standardized, evidence-based care protocols, participating in activities to improve emergency readiness and efficient care delivery. They also serve in an important educational role providing guidance and mentorship to peers, residents, and students. Quality of patient care, care delivery, and patient safety is enhanced with a GYNH as part of the OBGH team.

CLINICS CARE POINTS

- Gynecologic emergencies can be life-threatening, cause loss of fertility, and result in severe morbidity. As 24/7 onsite experts in care for acute gynecologic conditions, quality of patient care, care delivery, and patient safety are enhanced with a GYNH as part of the OBGH team.
- An OBGH must have expertise in acute, inpatient, obstetric, and gynecologic medicine.
- GYNHs provide 24/7 coverage for gynecologic needs in the hospital, improving efficiency in triage, admission, consultation, initiation of care plan, and discharge planning.
- GYNHs will commonly care for patients with acute gynecologic diagnoses such as pelvic pain, AUB, anemia, vaginal discharge, vulvar and labial masses, ectopic pregnancy, ovarian torsion, ovarian cyst rupture, vulvar abscess, missed/incomplete miscarriage, PUL, STI, pelvic inflammatory disease, and tubo-ovarian abscess.
- Procedures GYNHs may commonly perform include manual uterine evacuation at the bedside, dilation and curettage, and laparoscopy.
- Medical facilities desiring to implement a GYNH model must provide comprehensive support services. This includes diagnostic imaging, laboratory services, pharmacy stock and management of medications, surgical capabilities, and multispecialty consultative services.
- There is an urgent need for research regarding acute GYN conditions and optimal management. As experts in this field, GYNHs are well equipped and ideally positioned to contribute to this area. GYNHs should be engaged in quality improvement and research activities to advance the field such as the development of gynecologic medicine by researching, developing, and implementing protocols and order sets for standardization and optimization of care.
- GYNHs must be aware of facility-specific and system-specific gynecologic patient outcomes to target and guide implementation of necessary quality improvement initiatives.
- The GYNH can serve as the point person for educational activities for all learners in the hospital setting.

DISCLOSURE

J. Eaton has served on membership/advisory committee or review panels for Organon.

REFERENCES

1. McCue B. What is an obstetrics/gynecology hospitalist? Obstet Gynecol Clin North Am 2015;42(3):457–61.
2. McCue B, Fagnabnt R, Townsend A, et al. Definitions of obstetric and gynecologic hospitalists. Obstet Gynecol 2016;127(2):393–7.
3. Olson R, Garite TJ, Fishman A, et al. Obstetrician/gynecologist hospitalists: can we improve safety and outcomes for patients and hospitals and improve lifestyle for physicians? Am J Obstet Gynecol 2012;207(2):81–6.
4. Lawrence HC 3rd. New models of care. Clin Obstet Gynecol 2017;60(4):811–7.
5. Srinivas SK. Potential impact of obstetrics and gynecology hospitalists on safety of obstetric care. Obstet Gynecol Clin North Am 2015;42(3):487–91.
6. Yim GW, Park SJ, Lee EJ, et al. Impact of gynecologic hospitalist on patient waiting time at the emergency department in Korea: A retrospective pre-post cohort study. Taiwan J Obstet Gynecol 2021;60(5):851–6.
7. Kisuule F, Howell E. Hospitalists and their impact on quality, patient safety, and satisfaction. Obstet Gunecol Clin N Am 2015;42:433–46.
8. Swain C, Simon M, Monks B. Organizing an effective obstetric/gynecologic hospitalist program. Obstet Gynecol Clin North Am 2015;42(3):519–32.
9. American College of Obstetricians and Gynecologists' Committee on Patient Safety and Quality Improvement; American College of Obstetricians and Gynecologists' Committee on Obstetric Practice. Committee opinion no. 657 summary: the obstetric and gynecologic hospitalist. Obstet Gynecol 2016;127(2):419.
10. Patient safety in obstetrics and gynecology. ACOG Committee Opinion No. 447. American College of Obstetricians and Gynecologists. Obstet Gynecol 2009;114: 1424–7.
11. Kalinowska V, Huang Y, Alexander B, et al. Hospital volume and quality of care for emergency gynecologic care. Obstet Gynecol 2024;143(2):303–11.
12. Torbenson VE, Tatsis V, Bradley SL, et al. Use of obstetric and gynecologic hospitalists is associated with decreased severe maternal morbidity in the United States. J Patient Saf 2023;19(3):202–10.
13. Tessmer-Tuck J, McCue B. The ob/gyn hospitalist. contemporary OB/GYN. Available at: https://www.contemporaryobgyn.net/view/obgyn-hospitalist. [Accessed 8 December 2023].
14. Borhart J, Bavolek RA. Obstetric and gynecologic emergencies. Emerg Med Clin North Am 2019;37(2):xvii–xviii.
15. Fauconnier A, Provot J, Le Creff I, et al. A framework proposal for quality and safety measurement in gynecologic emergency care. Obstet Gynecol 2020;136(5):912–21.
16. Garber A, Rao PM, Rajakumar C, et al. Postpartum magnesium sulfate overdose: a multidisciplinary and interprofessional simulation scenario cureus: medical knowledge for the world. Cureus 2018;10(Issue 4):e2446.
17. Committee opinion no. 487: preparing for clinical emergencies in obstetrics and gynecology. Obstet Gynecol 2011;117(4):1032–4.
18. Subbe CP, Davies RG, Williams E, et al. Effect of introducing the Modified Early Warning score on clinical outcomes, cardio-pulmonary arrests and intensive care utilisation in acute medical admissions. Anaesthesia 2003;58(8):797–802.
19. Kripalini S, Pope A, Rask K, et al. Hospitalist as teachers: how do they compare to subspecialty and general medicine faculty? J Gen Intern Med 2004;19:8–15.
20. Torbenson VE, Riggan KA, Weaver AL, et al. Second victim experience among OBGYN trainees: what is their desired form of support? South Med J 2021; 114(4):218–22.

Periviability for the Ob-Gyn Hospitalist

Eesha Dave, MD, Katherine S. Kohari, MD, Sarah N. Cross, MD*

KEYWORDS

- Periviable birth • Extremely preterm birth • Neonatal palliative care
- Patient counseling • Termination

KEY POINTS

- The periviable period is defined as 20 0/7 to 25 6/7 weeks gestational age (GA).
- While extremely preterm neonatal outcomes have improved over the past few decades, there is still great uncertainty surrounding how individual neonates will fare in terms of overall survival and long-term morbidity.
- Understanding a patient's wishes and values is essential to counseling and caring for them. It is important to recognize that while some families may elect for neonatal resuscitation, others may elect for neonatal palliative care, or others may desire something else in between. Termination of pregnancy is appropriate to offer, depending on state laws and GA.
- Interdisciplinary care between obstetric and neonatal care teams is essential to optimizing outcomes. Depending on resources and hospital settings, transferring patients prior to delivery can help optimize outcomes for both mothers and neonates.

INTRODUCTION

Periviable birth is a medically and emotionally complicated event. The gestational ages (GAs) that comprise periviability have changed over the last several decades due to medical advances. However, there are still great variations in neonatal survival and outcomes during this fragile period. Additionally, the changing political-legal landscape is altering evidence-based options for patients delivering at extreme prematurity leading to increased maternal morbidity.[1] For these reasons, the management of individuals at risk for periviable birth involves both maternal and neonatal considerations. For some families faced with the possibility of a periviable birth, the decisions surrounding how to proceed may be very clear. However, given the great uncertainty

Division of Maternal Fetal Medicine, Department of Obstetrics, Gynecology and Reproductive Sciences, Yale School of Medicine, New Haven, CT, USA
* Corresponding author. Division of Maternal Fetal Medicine, Department of Obstetrics, Gynecology and Reproductive Sciences, Yale School of Medicine, 333 Ceder Street, New Heaven, CT 06520.
E-mail address: sarah.cross@yale.edu

Obstet Gynecol Clin N Am 51 (2024) 567–583
https://doi.org/10.1016/j.ogc.2024.05.008
0889-8545/24/© 2024 Elsevier Inc. All rights reserved, including those for text and data mining, AI training, and similar technologies.

in outcome, many families face decisional uncertainty. Management decisions do not rest solely on what can be done, but on patients' wishes for themselves and their future neonate. A detailed and nuanced discussion is therefore necessary between patient and provider to achieve shared-decision making.

HISTORIC CONSIDERATIONS & DEFINITIONS

The term periviability refers to a period of pregnancy in which post-natal survival is not definitely assured, especially as related to prematurity. While survivability is 0 at less than 20 weeks GA and close to 100% at 39 weeks GA, for infants born at the thresholds of viability, outcomes vary greatly.

Historic data on survivability are very interesting. Data on neonatal mortality between 1958 and 1969 did not include any data on infants born less than 25 weeks GA.[2] Overall in that study, survivability was not greater than 50% until 29 weeks GA.[2] Interventions such as antenatal corticosteroids, introduced in the 1970s, heralded a new era in the management and outcomes of preterm infants.[3] In updated studies from 1976 to 1979 and 1979 to 1982, 50% survivability had improved to approximately 27 weeks GA.[4–6] Data from the National Institute of Child Health and Human Development (NICHD) Neonatal Research Network, published in 1991 to 1992, reported a 50% survival rate at 24 weeks GA.[7] Updated NICHD data from 2003 to 2007 showed a 55% survival rate at 24 weeks GA.[8]

A joint workshop by the Eunice Kennedy Shriver NICHD, Society for Maternal-Fetal Medicine (SMFM), American Academy of Pediatrics, and American College of Obstetricians and Gynecologists (ACOG) opted to define periviable birth as those occurring between 20 0/7 and 25 6/7 weeks GA, as this reflected the GA range where survival ranged from 0 (at 20 weeks GA) to more than 50% (at 25 weeks GA).[9] This time frame is an intentional choice highlighting the evolution of management of periviable neonates.

In the United States (US) between 2014 and 2020 there has been a significant increase in the active treatment of live born neonates between 22 0/7 and 25 6/7 weeks GA,[10] likely owing to the increased likelihood for survival as compared to historic cohorts. However, the underlying reason for increased rates of active treatment are not clearly described and may reflect changing national political landscapes, as well as hospital policies around parental-decision making.

CLINICAL ETIOLOGIES AND PRESENTATIONS

Only a very small percentage of births, 0.4% to 0.5%, occur at or prior to 27 weeks GA. Yet, these births constitute over 40% of infant deaths, and further represent the majority of neonatal deaths.[9] ACOG reports that rates of preterm delivery have been increasing over the past few years. A prior history of preterm delivery is one of the primary risk factors for subsequent preterm birth.[11,12] A prior history of periviable delivery is associated with a recurrence of a periviable delivery, but is not a sensitive marker.[13]

Short cervix and cervical insufficiency are variables that also increase the risk of early delivery especially in the absence of interventions such as vaginal progesterone or cerclage placement. Other factors such as preterm labor and preterm premature rupture of membranes (PPROM) underlie about two-thirds of all periviable births.[11,13] Antepartum hemorrhage or abruption contributes to about a tenth of these births.[14] In contrast, iatrogenic preterm birth is rarer, but sometimes indicated in the periviable period, such as in the presence of severe preeclampsia or hemolysis, elevated liver enzymes, and low platelet syndrome (HELLP), which was reported in 4% of periviable deliveries.[11,13]

Some risk factors for preterm birth are modifiable, including low maternal pre-pregnancy weight (defined as a body mass index < 18.5), tobacco use, substance use, and short pregnancy interval. The effect of systemic racism is known to be associated with increased rates of preterm birth, with Black and Indigenous people having higher rates of early delivery. In 2019, the rate of spontaneous preterm birth for non-Hispanic Black people was 14.4% versus only 9.3% for White people.[15]

PATIENT COUNSELING

Counseling patients at risk for periviable birth is very challenging. There is often medical uncertainty, clinical acuity, time constraints, and most importantly, no set standard for management.[16] In fact, hospitals may have different thresholds for when resuscitation can be offered and when resuscitation must be offered.[14] These cut offs may be based on GA alone or may also include estimated fetal weight (EFW) thresholds. As a result, there is a large gray area with regards to the management of periviable birth.[16,17] Accurate and thorough counseling is challenging but also paramount for patient decision making.

First, physicians should make clear to patients that the authors' ability to predict survival, as well as outcomes in specific cases, while driven by data, are limited.[14] This is due to the factors that impact neonatal survival at such early GAs. Survival and outcomes in the periviable period are influenced by GA at birth, birth weight, neonatal sex, plurality, location of delivery, and administration of antenatal corticosteroids and magnesium sulfate.[16] As a result, it is important to offer all possible options to families with imminent periviable birth. Of note, these may differ based on GA and geographic location, and can include evaluation for neonatal resuscitation (also known as active treatment), palliative care or termination of pregnancy.[14]

Since GA is often the primary determinant of whether resuscitation is offered to patients and families, providers should obtain accurate, concrete information about how the pregnancy was dated.[16,17] Ideally, all patients have an ultrasound before 14 weeks as this most accurately confirms GA.[18] EFWs, which are most accurately determined by ultrasound in the periviable period, are also important when determining survival and long-term outcomes. Neonates with higher birth weights often have improved outcomes as compared to smaller counterparts.[8,19] The NICHD Extremely Preterm Birth Outcomes Tool is often used to quote chances of survival and morbidity to patients.[19] This calculator incorporates 5 variables including GA and EFW (**Fig. 1**).

Next, it is important to elucidate patient and family values. Management decisions in periviable deliveries are complex and difficult, and counseling should offer a discussion of all possible options for the neonate from attempts at resuscitation to palliative care and termination. The authors recommend beginning this process by asking open-ended questions to gauge the families' past experiences, future goals, and intentions for their neonate.[16,17] Shared-decision making has been associated with lower grief scores.[20] Ultimately, patients value being able to make the best decisions for their neonate, which are also concordant with their own belief and value systems.[21] In line with this, it is important for providers to recognize any biases they may have, and keep those in mind when counseling patients.[14,17] A study found that providers who identified as "pro-life" were more likely to offer and attempt resuscitation of periviable neonates than those that were not.[22]

While counseling patients, providers should avoid rigid statements such as: "Do you want everything done for your child?" and "Do you want nothing done?" as these do not appropriately reflect the complexities of periviable birth.[9] Additionally, it is important to emphasize that decisions can be fluid. This means that a decision that a family elects

Extremely Preterm Birth Outcomes Tool

Overview	Use the Tool	About the Data	References

Use the Tool

This tool provides a range of possible outcomes for infants born extremely preterm. The outcomes are based on data from infants born at specific U.S. hospitals between 2006 and 2012. "Hospital range" in the tool results represent outcomes for 80% of hospitals included in this study (10th to 90th percentiles). Please note that the tool describes outcomes for groups of infants with similar characteristics. It does not predict outcomes for any individual infant. Visit About the Data to learn more.

Please enter information available at the time of birth to use the tool.

Have feedback on the tool?

Email us with your ideas for improvement. Be sure to include your role/profession and how you used the tool. We cannot give medical advice or diagnoses.

* **Indicates required field**

*Gestational Age
(Best estimate in completed weeks)

Select ⇕

*Birth Weight
(from 401-1000 grams)

⇕

* Infant Sex

○ Male   ○ Female

* Singleton Birth

○ Yes   ○ No

* Antenatal Steroids

○ Yes   ○ No

Clear   Submit

Infants Receiving Active Treatment
Average Survival: -
Hospital Range: -

All Infants, Including Infants Not Actively Treated
Average Survival: -
Hospital Range: -

Outcomes At 18-26 Months' Corrected Age Among Infants Who Survive: (About the Data)

Profound Neurodevelopmental Impairment	Moderate-Severe Neurodevelopmental Impairment	Blindness	Deafness	Moderate-Severe Cerebral Palsy	Cognitive Developmental Delay
-	-	-	-	-	-

PLEASE NOTE: Information from this website is not intended to be the only basis for making care decisions for an individual infant, nor is it intended to be a definitive means of predicting infant outcomes. Users should keep in mind that every infant is an individual, and that factors beyond those described on this website influence infant survival and development.

Fig. 1. Extremely Preterm Birth Outcomes Tool, Pregnancy and Perinatology Branch. November 27, 2023. Updated 3/2/2020. Retrieved from: https://www.nichd.nih.gov/research/supported/EPBO/use.

for now can be re-evaluated later especially as they process additional information or clinical statuses change.[9] Furthermore, electing for some interventions does not signify that the family desires all interventions.[14] It is very reasonable, for example, that families may desire breathing support for their neonates, but decline chest compressions. Some pregnant patients may elect for steroid administration for their neonates, but decline a cesarean due to its high morbidity to them and subsequent pregnancies.[14]

Additionally, it is important to differentiate the data and information regarding neonatal survival and neonatal outcomes for patients during counseling. This is because families may value survival and long-term outcomes differently. For some individuals, survival may be paramount over all else. For others, understanding the quality of life their child may have may influence the decisions they make.[16,17] While studies discuss longer term neurodevelopmental outcomes for periviable neonates, they bundle outcomes into moderate and severe categories. It is important to recognize that individual families may consider moderate or severe disabilities differently than how they are defined by the medical literature. For example, behavioral disabilities are often considered "minor" disabilities, and hearing disabilities are considered "severe", but families may disagree about the severity of these.[9,17]

Also, providers are not required to provide interventions, which are considered futile. While this may be difficult for some patients to comprehend, it does protect providers, who recognize that the authors' medical abilities are limited and that not all interventions will be beneficial to all neonates (such as giving betamethasone for fetal prematurity at 20 weeks GA to a patient who will deliver prior to 22 weeks GA).[16]

In a systematic review of parental communication needs during perinatal counseling at extreme prematurity, Kharrat and colleagues found that parents who felt adequately involved in decision making experienced less doubt.[23] They found that families valued honesty and that they want to hear more than just statistics related to morbidity and mortality. The authors highlighted the importance of having multiple conversations. The theme of hope emerged as important to families and that families do not want to be repeatedly reminded about the potential for neurodevelopmental disability. The authors also note that nursing support was important to families; nurses were able to re-explain information, assess a family's understanding, and were seen as a source of support and hope.[23] Lastly, studies have shown that decisional conflict and decisional regret is inversely correlated to families' perception of shared-decision making.[20]

Data suggest that there is wide variability in what is covered in antenatal counseling and that it varies by specialty.[24] A variety of tools exist to help families and clinicians in perinatal counseling and decision making, including a digital decision aid.[25] Experts recommend that families be simultaneously counseled by obstetricians (OB) (Maternal-Fetal Medicine [MFM]) and neonatology[26] to effectively provide comprehensive cohesive information.[26]

CLINICAL MANAGEMENT

Management of patients at risk for delivery in the periviable period depends upon the GA, the etiology of the presentation and the patient's wishes regarding not only neonatal management but also their own management. The plan of care should be arrived upon via shared-decision making and updated as needed as the clinical picture changes. Management will also depend upon state laws regulating abortion, availability of providers to perform second trimester terminations,[27] hospital capability regarding neonatal resuscitation, the ability to transport to another facility with additional services, and availability of palliative services. The ACOG and the SMFM have a consensus document on periviable birth with general guidance regarding obstetric interventions for threatened and imminent periviable births (**Table 1**)[28] and there is updated guidance on the use of antenatal corticosteroids at 22 weeks from ACOG (**Table 2**).[29]

Less than 22 Weeks Gestational Age

Currently, neonatal assessment for resuscitation is not recommended at less than 22 0/7 weeks GA.[28] Therefore, interventions such as antenatal corticosteroids, tocolysis for preterm labor to allow for antenatal steroid administration, magnesium sulfate for

Table 1
General guidance regarding obstetric interventions for threatened and imminent periviable birth by best estimate of gestational age[a]

	20 0/7 wk to 21 6/7 wk	22 0/7 wk to 22 6/7 wk	23 0/7 wk to 23 6/7 wk	24 0/7 wk to 24 6/7 wk	25 0/7 wk to 25 6/7 wk
Neonatal assessment for resuscitation[a]	Not recommended 1A	Consider 2B	Consider 2B	Recommended 1B	Recommended 1B
Antenatal corticosteroids	Not recommended 1A	Not recommended 1A	Consider 2B	Recommended 1B	Recommended 1B
Tocolysis for preterm labor to allow for antenatal corticosteroid administration	Not recommended 1A	Not recommended 1A	Consider 2B	Recommended 1B	Recommended 1B
Magnesium sulfate for neuroprotection	Not recommended 1A	Not recommended 1A	Consider 2B	Recommended 1B	Recommended 1B
Antibiotics to prolong latency during expectant management of preterm PROM if delivery is not considered imminent	Consider 2C	Consider 2C	Consider 2B	Recommended 1B	Recommended 1B
Intrapartum antibiotics for group B streptococci prophylaxis[b]	Not recommended 1A	Not recommended 1A	Consider 2B	Recommended 1B	Recommended 1B
Cesarean delivery for fetal indication[c]	Not recommended 1A	Not recommended 1A	Consider 2B	Consider 1B	Recommended 1B

[a] Survival of infants born in periviable period is dependent on resuscitation and support. Between 22 wk and 25 wk of gestation, there may be factors in addition to gestational age that will affect the potential for survival and the determination of viability. Importantly, some families, concordant with their values and preferences, may choose to forgo such resuscitation and support. Many of the other decisions on this table will be linked to decisions regarding resuscitation and support and should be considered in that context.

[b] Group B streptococci carrier, or carrier status unknown.

[c] For example, persistently abnormal fetal heart rate patterns or biophysical testing, malpresentation.

From ACOG and SMFM Obstetric Care Consensus on Periviable Birth.[28]

	20 0/7 wk to 21 6/7 wk	22 0/7 wk to 22 6/7 wk	23 0/7 wk to 23 6/7 wk	24 0/7 wk to 24 6/7 wk	25 0/7 wk to 25 6/7 wk
Table 2 Updated guidance regarding antenatal corticosteroid administration for threatened and imminent periviable birth by best estimate of gestational age					
Antenatal corticosteroids	Not recommended 1A	Consider 2C	Consider 2B	Recommended 1B	Recommended 1B

Use of Antenatal Corticosteroids at 22 Weeks of Gestation. ACOG Practice Advisory from September 2021. American College of Obstetricians and Gynecologists and the Society for Maternal-Fetal Medicine in collaboration with Alison G. Cahill, MD, MSCI; Anjali J. Kaimal, MD, MAS; Jeffrey A. Kuller, MD; and Mark A. Turrentine, MD. Obstet Gynecol 2021.

fetal neuroprotection, intrapartum antibiotics for group B streptococci prophylaxis and cesarean delivery for fetal indications are not recommended at this GA.[28] If a patient is a candidate for expectant management at less than 22 0/7 weeks GA with PPROM, antibiotics to prolong latency can be considered.[28,30] In general, patients who are at risk for delivery at less than 22 0/7 weeks GA, but are otherwise stable, should be offered all options including expectant management with the hopes of arriving at a GA where neonatal assessment for resuscitation is possible, as well as abortion care, where available. Expectant management may not be advisable in some conditions such as preeclampsia with severe features with a contraindication to expectant management[31] or PPROM with chorioamnionitis,[30] then pregnancy interruption is recommended either via induction of labor or dilation and evaluation depending on patient's wishes and availability. At this time, the use of antenatal corticosteroids at less than 22 weeks GA is understudied and therefore not recommended,[32] but this is an area of active investigation.[33]

24 Weeks Gestational Age and Beyond

In general, neonatal assessment for resuscitation is recommended at 24 0/7 weeks GA and beyond.[28] It is important to note that neonatal assessment for resuscitation is not the same thing as neonatal resuscitation. After this assessment or once the resuscitation has started, the decision may be made not to continue. There may also be known antenatal factors where resuscitation will not be pursued in this period, such as severe fetal growth restriction (FGR) or major congenital anomalies where prematurity significantly changes the outcomes. In line with the general recommendation for neonatal assessment for resuscitation, at 24 0/7 weeks GA and beyond, obstetric interventions are generally recommended and may include antenatal corticosteroids, tocolysis for preterm labor to allow for antenatal steroid administration, magnesium sulfate for fetal neuroprotection, intrapartum antibiotics for group B streptococci prophylaxis, and antibiotics to prolong latency during expectant management of PPROM.[28] While cesarean delivery for fetal indications is recommended at 25 0/7 weeks GA and beyond, it can be considered between 24 0/7 and 24 6/7 weeks GA.[28]

22 to 23 Weeks Gestational Age

The period of 22 0/7 to 23 6/7 weeks GA is of greatest clinical equipoise due to the wide range of neonatal outcomes. Between 23 0/7 and 23 6/7 weeks GA, ACOG and SMFM recommend considering all obstetric interventions including neonatal assessment for resuscitation, antenatal corticosteroids, tocolysis for preterm labor to allow for antenatal steroid administration, magnesium sulfate for fetal neuroprotection, intrapartum antibiotics for group B streptococci prophylaxis, and antibiotics to prolong latency during expectant management of PPROM and cesarean delivery for fetal indications.[28] ACOG and SMFM encourage consideration of neonatal assessment for resuscitation and antibiotics to prolong latency during expectant management of PPROM between 22 0/7 and 22 6/7 weeks GA[28] and most recently adapted consideration of antenatal corticosteroids in this period.[32] There is mounting evidence that steroids at 22 weeks improve survival and neonatal outcomes.[33] Between 22 0/7 and 22 6/7 weeks GA tocolysis for preterm labor to allow for antenatal steroid administration, magnesium sulfate for fetal neuroprotection, intrapartum antibiotics for group B streptococci prophylaxis, and cesarean delivery for fetal indications are still not officially recommended,[28] but in practice are frequently performed when patients desire evaluation for neonatal resuscitation. Again, where available, patients may opt for abortion care rather than delivery or expectant management.

Cesarean Delivery

Patients desiring evaluation for neonatal resuscitation should be encouraged to receive obstetric interventions known to improve outcomes, such as neonatal corticosteroids. A related, but separate conversation should occur regarding mode of delivery given the increased morbidity for the pregnant person associated with cesarean delivery.[34,35]

While cesarean deliveries are increasing in the periviable period[36] patients should receive counseling on what the authors know regarding outcomes after cesarean delivery. There are no randomized controlled trial data to guide mode of delivery decisions in the periviable period. A review from 2013 concluded that data do not support routine cesarean to improve perinatal mortality or neurologic outcome in early preterm infants, but does appear to offer survival benefit to breech presenting fetuses, and may offer survival advantage to growth-restricted infants regardless of presentation.[37] Birth certificate data linked to infant death data show that cesarean delivery is associated with decreased odds of neonatal death and infant mortality in non-cephalic fetuses born at 22 to 28 weeks GA.[35] Looking specifically at 22 weeks GA, birth certificate data have shown cesarean delivery to be associated with higher rates of neonatal survival.[38]

Perinatal Palliative Care

There are increasing numbers of hospital centers offering perinatal palliative care programs. The option of perinatal palliative comfort care should be offered to families at risk for delivery in the periviable period.[39] The availability of these programs gives families a respectful option besides resuscitation. They focus on optimizing neonatal comfort at birth and in the newborn period.[28] Shared-decision making is critical to helping patients decide if perinatal palliative care is most in line with their values. Of note, the availability of palliative care may be influenced by a hospital's guidelines on neonatal resuscitation, GA, and overall assessment of fetal status or prognosis.[28,39]

Transport

If a patient at risk for periviable birth presents to a hospital without appropriate resources, a decision must be made about transport. If the patient is stable for transport, ideally they are transported prior to delivery. Transport may be indicated due to GA capabilities of the neonatal intensive care unit (NICU) or availability of maternal services such as a provider who can perform a dilation and evacuation (D&E). Decisions about what interventions to begin for transport should be made collaboratively with the patient and both the transporting and receiving care teams.

OUTCOMES
Fetal

Fetal risks in the periviable period mostly relate to a risk for fetal demise during a period of expectant management. In the EPIPAGE-2 study, which is a national prospective study of outcomes of PPROM at 22 to 25 weeks GA, there was an approximate 5% risk of fetal demise.[40]

Neonatal

The most important factor in neonatal survival and outcomes is the GA at birth.[19] There is an inverse relationship with neonatal morbidity and mortality and GA at delivery.[11] The second most important factor in neonatal survival is birth weight. The NICHD Extremely Preterm Birth Outcomes Tool also incorporates whether antenatal steroids were administered, singleton birth, and infant sex.[19] Survival is additionally impacted by whether infants receive active treatment (resuscitation). When looking at survival data, it is important to note whether the statistics are including all infants or only those that receive active treatment in the denominator. Data from 637 US centers in the Vermont Oxford Network looked at 45179 births from 2006 to 2012 and 25969 births from 2013 to 2016 showed an improvement in survival to hospital discharge (or 1 year of life if still hospitalized) amongst actively treated infants between 22 0/7 and 25 6/7 weeks GA (mean 24.1 weeks GA) across these cohorts from 66% to 70%.[41] In this study, there was an increase in actively treated infants at 22 weeks GA from 28% to 33% and an increase in observed survival from 21% to 25% amongst actively treated infants. At 23 weeks, there was an increase in actively treated infants from 82% to 88% and an increase in survival from 45% to 51%. At 24 weeks the rate of active treatment was 98% in the first cohort and 99% in the second, survival was 67% in the first cohort and 70%. At 25 weeks GA, the rate of active treatment was 99% in the first cohort and 100% in the second cohort and survival was 80% versus 83%. Interestingly, in this article incorporation of birth hospital into a model to predict outcome improved estimates of survival, which was especially pronounced at 22 and 23 weeks.[41]

Prematurity is associated with significant short- and long-term morbidity with risks inversely proportional to GA. In the EPIPAGE-2 study from France, which included 2205 births in 2011, survivors at 23 to 26 weeks GA had a 12.9% rate for severe intraventricular or intraparenchymal hemorrhage, 25.6% rate of severe bronchopulmonary dysplasia, 6% rate of severe retinopathy of prematurity, and a 5.1% rate of severe necrotizing enterocolitis.[42] For each of these conditions, rates were generally inversely related to GA.

The NICHD Neonatal Research Network looked at outcomes for 4274 infants born at 11 centers at 22 to 24 weeks GA over 3 epochs (2000–2003, 2004–2007, and 2008–2011). The percentage of infants who survived without neurodevelopmental impairment (measured at 18–22 months corrected age) increased from 16% in the first epoch to 20% in the third epoch. It is important to note, that these data included outcomes for all infants, not limited to only those who received active treatment.[43] Broken down by GA (across all epochs), assuming that all survivors received active treatment, survival without neurodevelopmental impairment was 5.4% at 22 weeks GA, 14.6% of infants born at 23 weeks GA, and 29.4% of infants born at 24 weeks GA amongst those who received active treatment.

Some of the most promising data on outcomes for extremely premature infants comes from Japan. In a study of 1057 infants born at 22 to 25 weeks GA at 48 tertiary centers as part of the Neonatal Research Network from 2003 to 2005, survival at

3 years was 36% at 22 weeks GA, 62.9% at 23 weeks GA, 77.1% at 24 weeks GA, and 85.2% at 25 weeks GA.[44] The study does not specifically indicate that all infants received active treatment, but all were planned admissions to the NICU, so the authors presume that all infants received active treatment. At 3 years, cognitive delay was seen in 27.9%, 32.2%, 50%, and 57.1% of those born at 25, 24, 23, and 22 weeks GA, respectively. Neurodevelopmental impairment was seen in 36.8%, 37.3%, 57%, and 52.2% of those born at 25, 24, 23, and 22 weeks GA, respectively. Lastly, profound neurodevelopmental impairment was seen in 17%, 16%, 39.5%, and 30.4% of those born at 25, 24, 23, and 22 weeks GA, respectively.[44]

Maternal

Maternal risks in the periviable period relate to risks of on-going pregnancy, specifically expectant management of the specific condition and delivery. For example, expectant management of preeclampsia with severe features or expectant management of PPROM. Compared to those having a term birth, those delivering in the periviable period have been found to have increased rates of adverse outcomes including transfusion, unplanned operative procedure, unplanned hysterectomy, uterine rupture, and intensive care unit admission.[45]

Indication for delivery

A case-control study of 174 individuals with previable PPROM (at 14–22 weeks GA) found that 1 in 7 pregnant people experience significant morbidity.[46] A retrospective cohort study looking at patients with PPROM between 14 0/7 and 23 6/7 weeks gestational found a 60.2% composite maternal morbidity rate in those undergoing expectant management versus 33.0% in those undergoing termination of pregnancy. Adjusted analysis showed expectant management to be associated with a 3.47 odds of composite maternal morbidity, or a relative risk of 1.91.[47] HELLP syndrome at less than 23 weeks has been found to have a 45% chance of serious complications for the pregnant individual including hepatic rupture, posterior reversible leukoencephalopathy, need for intubation, acute renal failure, and death.[48]

Mode of delivery

Cesarean delivery is associated with an increased incidence of severe maternal morbidity at very early GAs (22–28 weeks GA).[35] Compared with cesarean at term, preterm low transverse cesarean is associated with an increased rate of subsequent uterine rupture.[49] Specifically in the periviable period, cesarean delivery has been found to be associated with an increased rate of uterine rupture in a subsequent pregnancy, even after low transverse hysterotomy.[50] Additionally, cesarean in the periviable period have an increased incidence of classical hysterotomy compared to term cesareans.[50] In addition to uterine rupture, classical hysterotomy is known to be associated with increased risks in subsequent pregnancies such as blood transfusion and hysterectomy.[51] Furthermore, a history of classical hysterotomy eliminates the option for future vaginal birth requiring repeat cesareans[52] and requires late preterm or early-term deliveries [53] with the known associated risks of both.

Postpartum

In the postpartum period, those having an extremely preterm birth (£ 27 weeks GA) have higher rates (31%) of not using contraception compared to those delivering at later GAs (15%–16%). They also have decreased odds of using highly or moderately effective contraception, as well as user-independent methods compared to those having term births.[54] There is no set interpregnancy interval recommendation for women who experience periviable birth, and many women with extremely preterm births decline contraception because they hope to conceive again soon. However, short interpregnancy intervals (defined as <18 months) in general are associated with increased risk of preterm birth, low birth weight, and poorer outcomes in subsequent pregnancies.[54] As a result, discussing contraceptive options with this group of patients should not be overlooked.

Periviable birth has been found to be associated with an increased risk for both new onset and exacerbation of existing mental health disorders within 12 months postpartum.[55] Similarly, symptoms of post-traumatic stress disorder are high amongst bereaved parents after a periviable delivery.[56]

Preterm birth is strongly associated with subsequent development cardiovascular disease. In a national cohort study of all singleton births in Sweden from 1973 to 2015 looking at subsequent development of ischemic heart disease in the 10 years after delivery, while preterm birth was associated with an adjusted hazard ratio of 2.47 (95% CI 2.16–2.82), those with a very preterm birth (22–27 weeks GA) had the highest risk of 4.04 (95% CI 2.69–6.08).[57] In this same cohort, all-cause mortality was increased in the 10 years after delivery for those having a preterm birth with an adjusted hazard ratio of 1.73 (95% CI 1.61–1.87) and for those delivering at 22 to 27 weeks GA was even higher at 2.20 (95% CI 1.63–2.96).[58] In this study, several causes of mortality were identified including cardiovascular, respiratory, diabetes, and cancer.

Subsequent pregnancies

The data on outcomes of a subsequent pregnancy after a periviable birth are limited. Not surprisingly, when compared to those with an index vaginal birth, those with an index cesarean birth have an increased rate of uterine rupture in a subsequent pregnancy. They were also found to deliver earlier (35.9 vs 36.9 weeks GA) and have a lower birth weight infant (2736 vs 3014 g).[34]

CONTROVERSIES & CHALLENGES

Although care and management of patients at risk for delivery in the periviable period is exceedingly challenging, several specific challenges are worth mentioning.

Accuracy of Gestational Age Estimation

Previously cited guidelines use GA as the driving factor in managing extremely premature pregnancies.[28] However, determination of GA is imperfect.[18] While the first day of the last menstrual period (LMP) is traditionally the first step in estimating the expected date of delivery, this assumes a regular menstrual cycle of 28 days with ovulation occurring on the 14th day. And while there are data suggesting that first trimester ultrasound is more accurate in estimating the due date[59,60] LMP is still the primary method of estimating the due date in the US.[18] Redating is reserved for large discrepancies between LMP and ultrasound. Other countries, such as Canada, have moved to using ultrasound over LMP to establish the due date.[61] In an uncomplicated pregnancy, a difference of a day or 2 or even a week may have little clinical impact, but in pregnancies at risk for periviable delivery, the clinical management and counseling can be altered.

Many have argued for an approach that "moves beyond the GA" when making medical decisions for extremely premature infants.[62] Specifically, because of the known margin of error with GAs some have argued that complex decisions should not be based on GA alone.[63,64] This approach opens consideration of interventions at less than 22 weeks GA in select cases.

Restrictions on Abortion

While it is recommended to discuss the option of abortion care as an evidence-based approach for the management of pregnancies at risk for periviable birth[28] and despite the evidence that full availability of options minimizes adverse outcomes for the pregnant individual,[47] abortion care is not universally available in the US. The impact of abortion bans on patients in the periviable period has been described.[1] In September 2021 Texas passed Senate Bills 4 and 8, which prohibits a physician ending a pregnancy even in a maternal medical emergency, and bans abortions once fetal cardiac activity is identified, respectively. Nambiar and colleagues, sought to investigate the impact of these bills on morbidity for pregnant individuals presenting at less than 22 weeks GA with a medical indication for delivery (PPROM, preeclampsia with severe features or vaginal bleeding) without preterm labor.[1] They found that 57% of patients experienced serious maternal morbidity compared to 33% who elected immediate abortion care in states where this was available.[1]

Patients in need of abortion care may not have access to a provider who can perform a D&E, even in states, where it is legal. In a meta-analysis of 58 cases of HELLP syndrome at less than 23 weeks GA, 10 cesarean deliveries were performed, half of which were done at less than 22 weeks GA. Of the remaining 5, 1 was performed for the intention of termination and 1 was performed in the setting of a stillbirth and 3 had live births via cesarean.[48] These findings highlight the importance of adequate training and availability for providers in D&E.

Preeclampsia with Severe Features

The management of specific conditions warrants mention. In management of preeclampsia with severe features, a fetus without expectation for survival at the time of diagnosis (such as extreme prematurity) is considered a contraindication to expectant management.[31] This means that patients presenting at less than 22 weeks GA with preeclampsia with severe features should be recommended to undergo abortion care. As this is not legally available in all states, patient care is significantly varied, as mentioned earlier, resulting in disparity of care based upon geographic location.

Fetal Growth Restriction

The management of a pregnancy with FGR at risk for delivery in the periviable period is additionally challenging. Given that birth weight is an important prognostic factor, infants that are small for GA, in addition to being extremely premature have even more guarded outcomes. In 1 series of pregnancies with FGR, defined as abdominal circumference £ 3rd percentile, the survival rate for delivery at £ 28 weeks GA was 13%.[65] Based on a perinatal survival rate of 0% and 12% for FGR fetuses delivered at 22 to 23 and 24 to 25 weeks GA respectively, these authors suggest that the cut-off between previable and periviable may be dependent on EFW in addition to GA.[66] Ultrasound performed within 7 days of birth has been shown to have an 8.7% mean absolute percent error in small for GA infants.[67] However, while most ultrasound estimates were within 10% of actual birth weight, most were underestimates. Ultrasound has also been shown to have a less than 10% average absolute percent difference (9.4%) with birth weight in the periviable period.[68] Given the margin of error, although small, it is reasonable to question whether EFW should be the primary determinant for offering management options.

Implicit Bias and Training in Counseling

It is known that maternal factors, such as parity, intendedness of pregnancy, race, education, and age influence patient counseling recommendations.[69] At the same time, data suggest that obstetric physicians feel underprepared in breaking bad news with patients.[70] Simulation can be used to improve provider skill in perinatal counseling[71,72] hopefully minimizing the effect of bias.

Quality of Life

Lastly, perceptions about quality of life differ between health care professionals and families. Focus groups of adults who were born between 24 0/7 and 30 0/7 were asked to reflect on decision making at the limit of viability given their personal life experiences.[73] Amongst these individuals, quality of life was difficult to define, they were unsure who to determine what a good quality of life is and by whom it should be determined.[73] Thus, illustrating the ambiguity and degree of personalization in evaluation of the maternal and neonatal outcomes from periviable birth.

SUMMARY

The management of periviable pregnancies at risk for delivery is complicated and nuanced. Our aim in presenting the literature is to underscore that each case must be individualized as there is no singular way to manage these pregnancies. Due to high levels of uncertainty and variability surrounding periviable birth, management should be based on the objective data, the clinical scenario, and most importantly, the patient's wishes. This is an evolving field and practitioners are encouraged to consult the most up to date guidelines when caring for their patients.

CLINICS CARE POINTS

- It is important to establish and confirm a correct estimated due date prior to counseling patients at risk for periviable birth since treatment options and neonatal outcomes vary greatly by gestational age.
- Additionally, it is important to identify available hospital resources and discuss cases with Neonatology, if possible, to determine next best steps. Some circumstances may require patients to be transferred to hospitals that offer higher levels of care.
- The NICHD Extremely Preterm Birth Outcomes Tool is a helpful tool for patient counseling. It provides more detailed information on survival and morbidity based on fetal factors such as sex, gestational age, and weight.
- Currently, neonatal resuscitation is not recommended at gestational ages younger than 22 weeks 0 days. In turn, cesarean delivery for neonatal benefit is not recommended prior to this gestational age.

DISCLOSURE

The authors have nothing to disclose.

REFERENCES

1. Nambiar A, Patel S, Santiago-Munoz P, et al. Maternal morbidity and fetal outcomes among pregnant women at 22 weeks' gestation or less with complications in 2 Texas hospitals after legislation on abortion. Am J Obstet Gynecol 2022; 227(4):648–650 e1.
2. Lubchenco LO, Searls DT, Brazie JV. Neonatal mortality rate: relationship to birth weight and gestational age. J Pediatr 1972;81(4):814–22.

3. Farrell PM, Kotas RV. The prevention of hyaline membrane disease: new concepts and approaches to therapy. Adv Pediatr 1976;23:213–69.

4. Philip AG, Little GA, Polivy DR, et al. Neonatal mortality risk for the eighties: the importance of birth weight/gestational age groups. Pediatrics 1981;68(1):122–30.

5. Lamont RF, Dunlop PD, Crowley P, et al. Spontaneous preterm labour and delivery at under 34 weeks' gestation. Br Med J (Clin Res Ed) 1983;286(6363):454–7.

6. Mercer BM. Periviable Birth and the Shifting Limit of Viability. Clin Perinatol 2017; 44(2):283–6.

7. Fanaroff AA, Wright LL, Stevenson DK, et al. Very-low-birth-weight outcomes of the National Institute of Child Health and Human Development Neonatal Research Network, May 1991 through December 1992. Am J Obstet Gynecol 1995;173(5): 1423–31.

8. Stoll BJ, Hansen NI, Bell EF, et al. Neonatal outcomes of extremely preterm infants from the NICHD Neonatal Research Network. Pediatrics 2010;126(3):443–56.

9. Raju TNK, Mercer BM, Burchfield DJ, et al. Periviable birth: executive summary of a joint workshop by the Eunice Kennedy Shriver National Institute of Child Health and Human Development, Society for Maternal-Fetal Medicine, American Academy of Pediatrics, and American College of Obstetricians and Gynecologists. Obstet Gynecol 2014;123(5):1083–96.

10. Venkatesh KK, Lynch CD, Costantine MM, et al. Trends in Active Treatment of Live-born Neonates Between 22 Weeks 0 Days and 25 Weeks 6 Days by Gestational Age and Maternal Race and Ethnicity in the US, 2014 to 2020. JAMA 2022; 328(7):652–62.

11. Prediction and prevention of spontaneous preterm birth: ACOG practice bulletin summary, Number 234. Obstet Gynecol 2021;138(2):320–3.

12. Marinovich ML, Regan AK, Gissler M, et al. Associations between interpregnancy interval and preterm birth by previous preterm birth status in four high-income countries: a cohort study. BJOG 2021;128(7):1134–43.

13. Mercer B, Milluzzi C, Collin M. Periviable birth at 20 to 26 weeks of gestation: proximate causes, previous obstetric history and recurrence risk. Am J Obstet Gynecol 2005;193(3 Pt 2):1175–80.

14. ACOG. obstetric care consensus No. 3: periviable birth. Obstet Gynecol 2015; 126(5):e82–94.

15. Prediction and Prevention of Spontaneous Preterm Birth: ACOG Practice Bulletin. Number 234. Obstet Gynecol 2021;138(2):e65–90.

16. Arnolds M, Laventhal N. Perinatal Counseling at the Margin of Gestational Viability: Where We've Been, Where We're Going, and How to Navigate a Path Forward. J Pediatr 2021;233:255–62.

17. Haward MF, Gaucher N, Payot A, et al. Personalized Decision Making: Practical Recommendations for Antenatal Counseling for Fragile Neonates. Clin Perinatol 2017;44(2):429–45.

18. Committee Opinion No 700. Methods for Estimating the Due Date. Obstet Gynecol 2017;129(5):e150–4.

19. Extremely Preterm Birth Outcomes Tool. November 27. 2023. Available at: https://www.nichd.nih.gov/research/supported/EPBO. [Accessed 2 March 2020].

20. Geurtzen R, van den Heuvel JFM, Huisman JJ, et al. Decision-making in imminent extreme premature births: perceived shared decision-making, parental decisional conflict and decision regret. J Perinatol 2021;41(9):2201–7.

21. McDonnell S, Yan K, Kim UO, et al. Information order for periviable counseling: does it make a difference? J Pediatr 2021;235:100–106 e1.

22. Arzuaga BH, Meadow W. National variability in neonatal resuscitation practices at the limit of viability. Am J Perinatol 2014/05/27 2014;31(06):521–8.

23. Kharrat A, Moore GP, Beckett S, et al. Antenatal consultations at extreme prematurity: a systematic review of parent communication needs. J Pediatr 2018;196: 109–115 e7.

24. Tucker EB, McKenzie F, Panoch JE, et al. Comparing neonatal morbidity and mortality estimates across specialty in periviable counseling. J Matern Fetal Neonatal Med 2015;28(18):2145–9.

25. van den Heuvel JFM, Hogeveen M, Lutke Holzik M, et al. Digital decision aid for prenatal counseling in imminent extreme premature labor: development and pilot testing. BMC Med Inform Decis Mak 2022;22(1):7.

26. Kim BH, Feltman DM, Schneider S, et al. What Information Do Clinicians Deem Important for Counseling Parents Facing Extremely Early Deliveries?: Results from an Online Survey. Am J Perinatol 2023;40(6):657–65.

27. ACOG Practice Bulletin. No. 135: Second-trimester abortion. Obstet Gynecol 2013;121(6):1394–406.

28. Periviable birth. Obstetric Care Consensus No. 6. American College of Obstetricians and Gynecologists. Obstet Gynecol 2017;130:e187–99.

29. Use of Antenatal Corticosteroids at 22 Weeks of Gestation. ACOG Practice Advisory from September 2021. American College of Obstetricians and Gynecologists and the Society for Maternal-Fetal Medicine in collaboration with Alison G. Cahill, MD, MSCI; Anjali J. Kaimal, MD, MAS; Jeffrey A. Kuller, MD; and Mark A. Turrentine, MD. Obstet Gynecol 2021.

30. Siegler Y, Weiner Z, Solt I. ACOG Practice Bulletin No. 217: Prelabor Rupture of Membranes. Obstet Gynecol 2020;136(5):1061.

31. Gestational Hypertension and Preeclampsia: ACOG Practice Bulletin. Number 222. Obstet Gynecol 2020;135(6):e237–60.

32. Cahill AG, Kaimal AJ, Kuller JA, et al. Use of Antenatal Corticosteroids at 22 Weeks of Gestation. 2022. Available at: https://www.acog.org/clinical/clinical-guidance/practice-advisory/articles/2021/09/use-of-antenatal-corticosteroids-at-22-weeks-of-gestation. [Accessed 27 November 2023].

33. Battarbee AN. Antenatal Corticosteroids at 21-23 Weeks of Gestation. Obstet Gynecol 2023. https://doi.org/10.1097/AOG.0000000000005352.

34. Lannon SM, Guthrie KA, Reed SD, et al. Mode of delivery at periviable gestational ages: impact on subsequent reproductive outcomes. J Perinat Med 2013;41(6): 691–7.

35. Bitas C, Onishi K, Saade G, et al. Neonatal and maternal outcomes at 22-28 weeks of gestation by mode of delivery. Obstet Gynecol 2024;143(1):113–21.

36. Rossi RM, Hall E, DeFranco EA. Contemporary trends in cesarean delivery utilization for live births between 22 0/7 and 23 6/7 weeks of gestation. Obstet Gynecol 2019;133(3):451–8.

37. Mercer BM. Mode of delivery for periviable birth. Semin Perinatol 2013;37(6): 417–21.

38. Vidavalur R, Hussain Z, Hussain N. Association of Survival at 22 Weeks' Gestation With Use of Antenatal Corticosteroids and Mode of Delivery in the United States. JAMA Pediatr 2023;177(1):90–3.

39. Kaempf JW, Tomlinson MW, Tuohey J. Extremely premature birth and the choice of neonatal intensive care versus palliative comfort care: an 18-year single-center experience. J Perinatol 2016;36(3):190–5.

40. Lorthe E, Torchin H, Delorme P, et al. Preterm premature rupture of membranes at 22-25 weeks' gestation: perinatal and 2-year outcomes within a national

population-based study (EPIPAGE-2). Am J Obstet Gynecol 2018;219(3):298 e1–e298 e14.

41. Rysavy MA, Horbar JD, Bell EF, et al. Assessment of an Updated Neonatal Research Network Extremely Preterm Birth Outcome Model in the Vermont Oxford Network. JAMA Pediatr 2020;174(5):e196294.

42. Ancel PY, Goffinet F, Group EW. EPIPAGE 2: a preterm birth cohort in France in 2011. BMC Pediatr 2014;14:97.

43. Younge N, Goldstein RF, Bann CM, et al. Survival and Neurodevelopmental Outcomes among Periviable Infants. N Engl J Med 2017;376(7):617–28.

44. Ishii N, Kono Y, Yonemoto N, et al. Outcomes of infants born at 22 and 23 weeks' gestation. Pediatrics 2013;132(1):62–71.

45. Rossi RM, DeFranco EA. Maternal Complications Associated With Periviable Birth. Obstet Gynecol 2018;132(1):107–14.

46. Dotters-Katz SK, Panzer A, Grace MR, et al. Maternal Morbidity After Previable Prelabor Rupture of Membranes. Obstet Gynecol 2017;129(1):101–6.

47. Sklar A, Sheeder J, Davis AR, et al. Maternal morbidity after preterm premature rupture of membranes at <24 weeks' gestation. Am J Obstet Gynecol 2022; 226(4):558 e1–e558 e11.

48. Mossayebi MH, Iyer NS, McLaren RA Jr, et al. HELLP syndrome at <23 weeks' gestation: a systematic literature review. Am J Obstet Gynecol 2023;229(5): 502–515 e10.

49. Sciscione AC, Landon MB, Leveno KJ, et al. Previous preterm cesarean delivery and risk of subsequent uterine rupture. Obstet Gynecol 2008;111(3):648–53.

50. Lannon SMR, Guthrie KA, Vanderhoeven JP, et al. Uterine rupture risk after periviable cesarean delivery. Obstet Gynecol 2015;125(5):1095–100.

51. Thompson BB, Reddy UM, Burn M, et al. Maternal Outcomes in Subsequent Pregnancies After Classical Cesarean Delivery. Obstet Gynecol 2022;140(2): 212–9.

52. ACOG Practice Bulletin. No. 205: Vaginal Birth After Cesarean Delivery. Obstet Gynecol 2019;133(2):e110–27.

53. American College of O, Gynecologists' Committee on Obstetric Practice SfM-FM. Medically Indicated Late-Preterm and Early-Term Deliveries: ACOG Committee Opinion, Number 831. Obstet Gynecol 2021;138(1):e35–9.

54. Robbins CL, Farr SL, Zapata LB, et al. Postpartum contraceptive use among women with a recent preterm birth. Am J Obstet Gynecol 2015;213(4):508 e1–e9.

55. Bruno AM, Horns JJ, Allshouse AA, et al. Association Between Periviable Delivery and New Onset of or Exacerbation of Existing Mental Health Disorders. Obstet Gynecol 2023;141(2):395–402.

56. Tucker EB, Laitano T, Hoffman SM, et al. The impact of decision quality on mental health following periviable delivery. J Perinatol 2019;39(12):1595–601.

57. Crump C, Sundquist J, Howell EA, et al. Pre-Term Delivery and Risk of Ischemic Heart Disease in Women. J Am Coll Cardiol 2020;76(1):57–67.

58. Crump C, Sundquist J, Sundquist K. Preterm delivery and long term mortality in women: national cohort and co-sibling study. BMJ 2020;370:m2533.

59. Savitz DA, Terry JW Jr, Dole N, et al. Comparison of pregnancy dating by last menstrual period, ultrasound scanning, and their combination. Am J Obstet Gynecol 2002;187(6):1660–6.

60. Butt K, Lim KI. Guideline No. 388-Determination of Gestational Age by Ultrasound. J Obstet Gynaecol Can 2019;41(10):1497–507.

61. Your Pregnancy - Routine Ultrasound. Available at: https://www.pregnancyinfo. ca/your-pregnancy/routine-tests/ultrasound/. [Accessed 1 January 2024].

62. Tyson JE, Parikh NA, Langer J, et al. Intensive care for extreme prematurity–moving beyond gestational age. N Engl J Med 2008;358(16):1672–81.
63. De Proost L, Ismaili M, hamdi H, et al. On the limits of viability: toward an individualized prognosis-based approach. J Perinatol 2020;40(12):1736–8.
64. Mercurio MR, Carter BS. Resuscitation policies for extremely preterm newborns: finally moving beyond gestational age. J Perinatol 2020;40(12):1731–3.
65. Lawin-O'Brien AR, Dall'Asta A, Knight C, et al. Short-term outcome of periviable small-for-gestational-age babies: is our counseling up to date? Ultrasound Obstet Gynecol 2016;48(5):636–41.
66. Dall'Asta A, Penas Da Costa MA, Sorrentino S, et al. Counseling in Fetal Medicine: pre- and periviable fetal growth restriction. Ultrasound Obstet Gynecol 2023. https://doi.org/10.1002/uog.27519.
67. Blumenfeld YJ, Lee HC, Pullen KM, et al. Ultrasound estimation of fetal weight in small for gestational age pregnancies. J Matern Fetal Neonatal Med 2010;23(8):790–3.
68. Ethridge JK Jr, Louis JM, Mercer BM. Accuracy of fetal weight estimation by ultrasound in periviable deliveries. J Matern Fetal Neonatal Med 2014;27(6):557–60.
69. Kunkel MD, Downs SM, Tucker Edmonds B. Influence of Maternal Factors in Neonatologists' Counseling for Periviable Pregnancies. Am J Perinatol 2017;34(8):787–94.
70. Gueneuc A, Dagher C, Rameh G, et al. Announcing fetal pathology: Challenges encountered by physicians and potential role of simulation in training for breaking bad news. J Gynecol Obstet Hum Reprod 2021;50(4):102044.
71. Boss RD, Donohue PK, Roter DL, et al. "This is a decision you have to make": using simulation to study prenatal counseling. Simul Healthc 2012;7(4):207–12.
72. Tucker EB, McKenzie F, Panoch J, et al. Evaluating shared decision-making in periviable counseling using objective structured clinical examinations. J Perinatol 2019;39(6):857–65.
73. de Boer A, De Proost L, de Vries M, et al. Perspectives of extremely prematurely born adults on what to consider in prenatal decision-making: a qualitative focus group study. Arch Dis Child Fetal Neonatal Ed 2023. https://doi.org/10.1136/archdischild-2023-325997.

Printed and bound by CPI Group (UK) Ltd, Croydon, CR0 4YY

08/05/2025

01864750-0006